GnRH Analogues in Reproduction and Gynecology

DEDICATION

We dedicate this book to the Organizing Committee: E. Johannison, P. Melzer, H.S. Jacobs, P.C. Sizonenko, F.H. Schroder and F. Comite and to all our colleagues whose work with GnRH analogues is increasing the quality of life for individuals suffering the wide range of medical conditions benefited by the use of these agents.

B. H. Vickery
B. Lunenfeld

GnRH ANALOGUES IN CANCER AND HUMAN REPRODUCTION

VOLUME II

GnRH Analogues in Reproduction and Gynecology

Edited by

B. H. Vickery and B. Lunenfeld

KLUWER ACADEMIC PUBLISHERS
DORDRECHT / BOSTON / LONDON

Distributors

for the United States and Canada: Kluwer Academic Publishers, PO Box 358, Accord Station, Hingham, MA 02018-0358, USA
for all other countries: Kluwer Academic Publishers Group, Distribution Center, PO Box 322, 3300 AH Dordrecht, The Netherlands

British Library Cataloguing in Publication Data

GnRH analogues in cancer and human reproduction.
Vol.2. GnRH analogues in reproduction and gynecology.
1. Women. Reproductive system. Cancer. Drug therapy
I. Vickery, B. H. (Brian H.), *1941-* II. Lunenfeld, Bruno
616.99'465061

ISBN-13: 978-94-010-6809-3 e-ISBN-13: 978-94-009-0721-8
DOI: 10.1007/978-94-009-0721-8

Library of Congress Cataloging-in-Publication Data

GnRH analogues in cancer and human reproduction / edited by B.H. Vickery and B. Lunenfeld
p. cm.
Includes bibliographical references.
Contents: Vol. 1. Basic aspects – v. 2. GnRH analogues in reproduction and gynecology – v. 3. Benign and malignant tumours – v. 4. Precocious puberty, contraception, safety issues.

1. Generative organs--Diseases--Hormone therapy--Congresses. 2. Luteinizing hormone releasing hormone--Derivatives--Therapeutic use--Congresses. 3. Generative organs--Cancer--Hormone therapy--Congresses. I. Vickery, Brian H., 1941- . II. Lunenfeld, Bruno.
[DNLM: 1. Neoplasms--drug therapy. 2. Pituitary Hormone Releasing Hormones--physiology. 3. Reproduction--drug effects. WK 515 G572]
RC877.G57 1989
618'.0461--dc20
DNLM/DLC
for Library of Congress 89-24592
CIP

Published in the United Kingdom by Kluwer Academic Publishers, PO Box 55, Lancaster, UK.

Kluwer Academic Publishers BV incorporates the publishing programmes of D. Reidel, Martinus Nijhoff, Dr W. Junk and MTP Press.

CONTENTS

CONTENTS OF OTHER VOLUMES

Volume I. Basic Aspects

Volume III. Benign and Malignant Tumors

Volume IV. Precocious Puberty, Contraception, Safety Issues

PREFACE

These four volumes comprising "GnRH Analogues in Cancer and Human Reproduction" are a distillation of the presentations of the invited speakers at a landmark International Symposium bearing the same name, organized by one of us (B.L.) and held in Geneva, Switzerland in February 1988. The Symposium was truly interdisciplinary spanning gonadal hormone dependent disease including various forms of cancer and ranging to control of fertility, both pro- and conception. The international flavor can be caught from the 480 participants and 259 contributors drawn from 14 countries. The Symposium, and therefore this book, would not have been possible without the backing of The International Committee for Research in Reproduction and the sponsorship of the International Society of Gynecologic Endocrinology, The Swiss Society of Fertility and Sterility, The University of Geneva School of Medicine, The Swiss Society of Endocrinology and The US Foundation for Studies in Reproduction Inc., and help from the World Health Organization.

B. H. Vickery
B. Lunenfeld
June 1989

LIST OF CONTRIBUTORS
TO THE SERIES

A. Abbondante
First Institute of Obstetrics and Gynecology
University "La Sapienza"
Rome, Italy

P. Abel
Department of Urology
Hammersmith Hospital
DuCane Road
London W12 OHS, UK

H. Abramovici
Departments of Obstetrics and Gynecology
Rambam Medical Center and Carmel Hospital, Technion
Israel Institute of Technology
Haifa 31096, Israel

V. Aleandri
First Institute of Obstetrics and Gynecology
University "La Sapienza"
Rome, Italy

Michel L. Aubert
Department of Pediatrics and Genetics
Division of Biology of Growth and Reproduction
University of Geneva Medical School
1211 Geneva 4, Switzerland

Tom M. Badger
Reproductive Endocrine Unit
Vincent Memorial Research Laboratories
Boston, MA 02114, USA

Sandor Bajusz
Veterans Administration Medical Center
1601 Perdido Street
New Orleans, LA 71046, USA

P. Barriere
IVF Department
CHU Nantes
44035-Nantes Cedex 01, France

H. Bartermann
Urologische Universitatsklinik Kiel
Arnold-Heller Strasse 7
D-2300 Kiel 1, FRG

M. Bartholomew
Department of Medicine/Endocrinology
Milton S. Hershey Medical Center
Pennsylvania State University
PO Box 850, Hershey, PA 17033, USA

D. Beck
Departments of Obstetrics and Gynecology
Ramban Medical Center and Carmel Hospital, Technion
Israel Institute of Technology
Haifa 31096, Israel

G. Benagiano
First Institute of Obstetrics and Gynecology
University "La Sapienza"
Rome, Italy

G. Bender
Department of Obstetrics and Gynecology
Staedtische Kliniken
Grafenstrasse 9
D-6100 Darmstadt, FRG

Z. Ben-Rafael
Interdepartmental Unit of Human Reproduction
Department of Obstetrics and Gynecology
The Chaim Sheba Medical Center and Sackler School of Medicine
Tel-Hashomer 52621, Israel

M. Berezin
Institute of Endocrinology
The Chaim Sheba Medical Center
Tel-Hashomer 52621, Israel

G. Bettendorf
UKE Frauenklinik
Division of Endocrinology
Martinistrasse 52
2000 Hamburg 20, FRG

Zvi Binor
Section of Reproductive Endocrinology/Infertility
Department of Obstetrics and Gynecology
Rush Medical College
Chicago, IL 60612, USA

W.P. Black
University Department of Obstetrics and Gynaecology
Glasgow Royal Infirmary
Glasgow G31 2ER, UK

J. Blankstein
Interdepartmental Unit of Human Reproduction
Department of Obstetrics and Gynecology
The Chaim Sheba Medical Center and Sackler School of Medicine
Tel-Hashomer 52621, Israel

Robert M. Blizzard
Department of Pediatrics
University of Virginia Medical School
PO Box 386
Charlottesville, VA 22901, USA

Zeev Blumenfeld
Departments of Obstetrics and Gynecology
Ramban Medical Center and Carmel Hospital
Technion, Israel Institute of Technology
Haifa 31096, Israel

Paul A. Boepple
Reproductive Endocrine Unit
Massachusetts General Hospital
Rear Blossom Street
Boston, MA 02114, USA

L. Boubli
Gynecologie-Obstetrique
Hopital Michel Levy, Annexe Conception
84a Rue de Lodi
13281 Marseille Cedex 6, France

A. Boucher
Department of Medicine/Endocrinology
Milton S. Hershey Medical Center
Pennsylvania State University
PO Box 850, Hershey, PA 17033, USA

Cyril Bowers
Endocrine Unit
Tulane University School of Medicine
New Orleans, LA 70112, USA

W. Braendel
UKE Frauenklinik
Division of Endocrinology
Martinistrasse 52
2000 Hamburg 20, FRG

J.M. Brandes
Departments of Obstetrics and Gynecology
Ramban Medical Center and Carmel Hospital, Technion
Israel Institute of Technology
Haifa 31096, Israel

R. Brauner
Unit of Pediatric Endocrinology and Diabetes
Hospital des Enfants Malades
75015 Paris, France

M. Breckwoldt
Department of Obstetrics and Gynecology
Division of Clinical Endocrinology
University of Freiburg
D-7800 Freiburg-im-Breisgau, FRG

Th. Bremen
Department of Obstetrics and Gynecology
Staedtische Kliniken
Grafenstrasse 9
D-6100 Darmstadt, FRG

Todd D. Brodie
Reproductive Endocrine Unit
Vincent Memorial Research Laboratories
Boston, MA 02114, USA

I.A. Brosens
Laboratory for Gynaecological Physiopathology
UZ Gasthuisberg
KU Leuven, Belgium

Robert Browneller
Abbott Laboratories
Abbott Park, IL 60064, USA

S.K. Burt
Pharmaceutical Discovery Division
Abbott Laboratories
Abbott Park, IL 60064, USA

Eugene N. Bush
Pharmaceutical Discovery Division
Abbott Laboratories
Abbott Park, IL 60064, USA

M. Camus
Center for Reproductive Medicine
Medical Campus, Vrije University Brussel
Laarbeeklaan 101
1090 Brussels, Belgium

R.J. Capetola
Ortho Pharmaceutical Corporation
Route 202
Raritan, NJ 08869, USA

R. Caplan
Department of Medicine/Endocrinology
Milton S. Hershey Medical Center
Pennsylvanian State University
PO Box 850, Hershey, PA 71033, USA

M. Carter
University Department of Obstetrics and Gynaecology
Glasgow Royal Infirmary
Glasgow G31 2ER, UK

E. Caspi
Department of Obstetrics and Gynecology
Assaf Harofe Medical Center
Zerefin, Israel

B. Charbonnel
IVF Department
CHU Nantes
44035-Nantes Cedex 01, France

J.L. Chaussain
Foundation de Recherche en Homonologie
PB110
94268 Fresnes Cedex, France

Claudia Chillik
Department of Obstetrics and Gynecology
Eastern Virginia Medical School
Norfolk, VA 23507, USA

Jean Cohen
Clinique Marignan
3 rue Marignan
75008 Paris, France

Ana Maria Comaru-Schally
Veterans Administration Medical Center
1601 Perdido Street
New Orleans, LA 70146, USA

Florence Comite
Department of Medicine and Gynecology
Yale University School of Medicine
New Haven, CT 06510-8063, USA

C. Conaghan
University Department of Obstetrics and Gynaecology
Glasgow Royal Infirmary
Glasgow G31 2ER, UK

P. Michael Conn
Department of Pharmacology
University of Iowa College of Medicine
Iowa City, IO 52242, USA

Angelo Conti
Ch. de Mornex 6
1003 Lausanne, Switzerland

F. Cornillie
Laboratory for Gynaecological Pathophysiology
UZ Gasthuisberg
KU Leuven, Belgium

R.M. Couch
Department of Pediatrics and Pathology
University of British Columbia
BC's Children's Hospital
Vancouver, BC V6H 3V4, Canada

J.R.T. Coutts
University Department of Obstetrics and Gynaecology
Glasgow Royal Infirmary
Glasgow G31 2ER, UK

J. Cox
Department of Urology
Central Middlesex Hospital
London, UK

John D. Crawford
Children's Service
Massachusetts General Hospital
Fruit Street
Boston, MA 02114, USA

John F. Crigler, Jr.
Department of Medicine
Division of Endocrinology, Children's Hospital
300 Longwood Avenue
Boston, MA 02115, USA

William F. Crowley Jr.
Departments of Medicine and Gynecology
Massachusetts General Hospital
Boston, MA 02114, USA

Lionel Cusan
Department of Molecular Endocrinology
Laval University Medical Center
Quebec G1V 4G2, Canada

Douglas R. Danforth
Department of Obstetrics and Gynecology
Eastern University Medical School
Norfolk, VA 23507, USA

F. Calais da Silva
A.Z. Middelheim
Antwerp 2020, Belgium

Adi Davidson
Interdepartmental Unit of Human Reproduction
Department of Obstetrics and Gynecology
The Chaim Sheba Medical Center and Sackler School of Medicine
Tel-Hashomer 52621, Israel

R. Deghenghi
Debiopharm SA
1003 Lausanne, Switzerland

F.H. de Jong
Department of Medicine II and Clinical Endocrinology
Erasmus University
Rotterdam, The Netherlands

L. Denis
A.Z. Middelheim
Antwerp 2020, Belgium

M. De Pauw
A.Z. Middelheim
Antwerp 2020, Belgium

J. De Schacht
Center for Reproductive Medicine
Medical Campus, Vrije Universiteit Brussel
Laarbeeklaan 101
1090 Brussels, Belgium

P. Devroey
Center for Reproductive Medicine
Medical Campus, Vrije Universiteit Brussel
Laarbeeklaan 101
1090 Brussels, Belgium

Gilbert Diaz
Pharmaceutical Discovery Division
Abbott Laboratories
Abbott Park, IL 60064, USA

M. Dirnfeld
Departments of Obstetrics and Gynecology
Ramban Medical Center and Carmel Hospital, Technion
Israel Institute of Technology
Haifa 31096, Israel

W. Paul Dmowski
Section of Reproductive Endocrinology/Infertility
Department of Obstetrics and Gynecology
Rush Medical College
Chicago, IL 60612, USA

Joshua Dor
Interdepartmental Unit of Human Reproduction
Department of Obstetrics and Gynecology
The Chaim Sheba Medical Center and Sackler School of Medicine
Tel-Hashomer 52621, Israel

J. Drago
Department of Medicine/Endocrinology
Milton S. Hershey Medical Center
Pennsylvania State University
PO Box 850, Hershey, PA 17033, USA

S.L.S. Drop
Sophia Children's Hospital
160 Gordelweg
3038 GE Rotterdam, The Netherlands

André Dupont
Department of Molecular Endocrinology
Laval University Medical Center
Quebec G1V 4G2, Canada

Anand S. Dutta
Pharmaceutical Division
Imperial Chemical Industries plc
Mereside, Alderley Park
Macclesfield, Cheshire SK10 4TG, UK

L. Edwards
Westminster Hospital
London SW1 2AP, UK

Adreian Elenbogen
Interdepartmental Unit of Human Reproduction
Department of Obstetrics and Gynecology
The Chaim Sheba Medical Center and Sackler School of Medicine
Tel-Hashomer 52621, Israel

D. Elia
Clinique Marignan
3 rue Marignan
75008 Paris, France

Jean Emond
Laval University Medical Center
Quebec G1V 4G2, Canada

G. Emons
Klinik für Franenheilkunde und Geburtshilfe
Institute für Biochemische Endokrinologie
Medizurische Universiteit zu Lübeck
D-2400 Lübeck, FRG

K. Engelbart
Hoechst AG
D-6230 Frankfurt 80, FRG

R. Erny
Gynecologie-Obstetrique
Hospital Michael Levy, Annexe Conception
84a rue de Lodi
13281 Marseille Cedex 6, France

N. Farah
Department of Urology
Central Middlesex Hospital
London, UK

S. Finnie
University Department of Obstetrics and Gynaecology
Glasgow Royal Infirmary
Glasgow G31 2ER, UK

J. Fleming
Department of Urology
Central Middlesex Hospital
London, UK

R. Fleming
University Department of Obstetrics and Gynaecology
Glasgow Royal Infirmary
Glasgow G31 2ER, UK

J.A. Foekens
Division of Endocrine Oncology
Rotterdam Cancer Institute
The Dr. Daniel den Hoed Cancer Center, Groene Hilledijk 301
3075 EA Rotterdam, The Netherlands

I. Fogelman
Department of Nuclear Medicine
Guy's Hospital
London, UK

Karl Folkers
Institute for Biomedical Research
The University of Texas at Austin
Austin, TX 78712, USA

C. Fouprie
Foundation de Recherche en Hormonologie
PB110
94268 Fresnes Cedex, France

R. Francois
Foundation de Recherche en Hormonologie
PB110
94268 Fresnes Cedex, France

Andrew J. Friedman
Brigham and Women's Hospital
Fertility and Endocrine Unit
75 Francis Street
Boston, MA 02115, USA

Barrington J.A. Furr
Bioscience I. Department
ICI Pharmaceuticals plc
Alderley Park, Macclesfield
Cheshire SK10 4TG, UK

F. Geisthövel
Department of Obstetrics and Gynecology
Division of Clinical Endocrinology
University of Freiburg
D-7800 Freiburg-im-Breisgau, FRG

B. Gilks
Department of Pediatrics and Pathology
University of British Columbia
BC's Children's Hospital
Vancouver BC V6H 3V4, Canada

L. Glode
Department of Medicine/Endocrinology
Milton S. Hershey Medical Center
Pennsylvania State University
PO Box 850, Hershey, PA 17033, USA

A. Golan
Department of Obstetrics and Gynecology
Assaf Harofe Medical Center
Zerefin, Israel

Jessie C. Goodpasture
Institute of Biological Sciences
Syntex Research
3401 Hillview Avenue
Palo Alto, CA 94304, USA

R. Gordon
Department of Medicine/Endocrinology
Milton S. Hershey Medical Center
Pennsylvania State University
PO Box 850, Hershey, PA 17033, USA

Jonathan Greer
Pharmaceutical Discovery Division
Abbott Laboratories
Abbott Park, IL 60064, USA

Melvin M. Grumbach
Department of Pediatrics
University of California San Francisco
San Francisco, CA 94943, USA

F. Hadziselimovic
Children's Hospital Basle
Römergasse 8
CH-4005 Basle, Switzerland

D.W. Hahn
Ortho Pharmaceutical Corporation
Route 202
Raritan, NJ 08869, USA

M. Hahn
Hoechst AG
D-6230 Frankfurt 80, FRG

H. Halkin
Institute of Endocrinology
The Chaim Sheba Medical Center
Tel-Hashomer 52621, Israel

Janet E. Hall
Reproductive Endocrine Unit
Vincent Memorial Research Laboratories
Boston, MA 02114, USA

M.P.R. Hamilton
University Department of Obstetrics and Gynaecology
Glasgow Royal Infirmary
Glasgow G31 2ER, UK

H. Harvey
Department of Medicine/Endocrinology
Milton S. Hershey Medical Center
Pennsylvania State University
PO Box 850, Hershey, PA 17033, USA

Fortuna Haviv
Pharmaceutical Discovery Division
Abbott Laboratories
Abbott Park, IL 60064, USA

M.J. Haxton
University Department of Obstetrics and Gynaecology
Glasgow Royal Infirmary
Glasgow G31 2ER, UK

D.L. Healey
Medical Research Center
Monash Medical Center
Prince Henry's Hospital Campus
Melbourne, Australia

A. Herman
Department of Obstetrics and Gynecology
Assaf Harofe Medical Center
Zerefin, Israel

P. Heuschen
Department of Obstetrics and Gynecology
Staedtische Kliniken
Grafenstrasse 9
D-6100 Darmstadt, FRG

P.C. Ho
Department of Obstetrics and Gynecology
University of Hong Kong
Hong Kong

Gary D. Hodgen
Jones Institute for Reproductive Medicine
Eastern University Medical School
Norfolk, VA 23507, USA

J.C. Huber
1st Department of Gynecology and Obstetrics
A-1090 Vienna, Austria

Magdalen E. Hull
Division of Reproductive Endocrinology
Department of Obstetrics and Gynecology
State University of New York at Stony Brook School of Medicine
Stony Brook, NY 11794-8091, USA

R. Hummelink
Sophia Children's Hospital
160 Gordelweg
3038 GE Rotterdam, The Netherlands

F.G. Hutchinson
Pharmaceutical Department, ICI Pharmaceutical plc
Alderley Park, Macclesfield
Cheshire SK10 4TG, UK

Vaclav Insler
Endocrinology Laboratory, Soroka Medical Center and
Division of Obstetrics and Gynecology
Clinical Biochemistry Unit, Faculty of Health Sciences
Ben-Gurion University of the Negev
Beer-Sheba 84101, Israel

Joseph Itskovitz
Department of Obstetrics and Gynecology
Eastern University Medical School
Norfolk, VA 23507, USA

M.E. Jamieson
University Department of Obstetrics and Gynaecology
Glasgow Royal Infirmary
Glasgow G31 2ER, UK

G. Jerabek-Sandow
Hoechst AG
D-6230 Frankfurt 80, FRG

Edwin S. Johnson
Pharmaceutical Discovery Division
Abbott Laboratories
Abbott Park, IL 60064, USA

W. Jäger
Department of Gynecology and Obstetrics
University of Erlangen-Nürnberg
8520 Erlangen, FRG

Themis Kamilaris
Division of Endocrinology
Vanderbilt University School of Medicine
Nashville, TN 37232, USA

Selna L. Kaplan
Department of Pediatrics
University of California San Francisco
San Francisco, CA 94943, USA

R. Kauli
Institute of Pediatric and Adolescent Endocrinology
Sackler Faculty of Medicine
Tel Aviv University
Tel Aviv, Israel

Daniel Kenigsberg
Division of Reproductive Endocrinology
Department of Obstetrics and Gynecology
State University of New York at Stony Brook School of Medicine
Stony Brook, NY 11794-8091, USA

F. Keuppens
A.Z. Middelheim
Antwerp 2020, Belgium

I. Khan
Center for Reproductive Medicine
Medical Campus, Vrije Universitiet Brussel
Laarbeeklaan 101
1090 Brussels, Belgium

Ludwig Kiesel
Division of Gynecological Endocrinology
Department of Obstetrics and Gynecology
University of Heidelberg
D-6900 Heidelberg, FRG

S. Kille
Hoechst AG
D-6230 Frankfurt 80, FRG

H. Kitson
Department of Pediatrics and Pathology
University of British Columbia
BC's Children's Hospital
Vancouver BC V6H 3V4, Canada

Jan G.M. Klijn
Division of Endocrine Oncology
Rotterdam Cancer Institute
The Dr. Daniel den Hoed Cancer Center, Groene Hilledijk 301
3075 EA Rotterdam, The Netherlands

Jasna Knezvic
Department of Pediatrics
University of California San Francisco
San Francisco, CA 94943, USA

R. Knuppen
Klinik für Biochemische Endokrinologie
Medizurische Universiteit zu Lübeck
D-2400 Lübeck, FRG

B. Krauss
Hoechst AG
D-6230 Frankfurt 80, FRG

Renee Kreuter
Department of Pediatrics and Genetics
Division of Biology of Growth and Reproduction
University of Geneva Medical School
1211 Geneva 4, Switzerland

Fernand Labrie
Department of Molecular Endocrinology
Laval University Medical Center
Quebec G1V 4G2, Canada

Yves Lacourciere
Laval University Medical Center
Quebec G1V 4G2, Canada

N. Lahlou
Foundation de Recherche en Hormonologie
PB110
94268 Fresnes Cedex, France

N. Lang
Department of Gynecology and Obstetrics
University of Erlangen-Nürnberg
8520 Erlangen, FRG

Zvi Laron
Beilinson Medical Center
Petah Tikva 49100, Israel

André Lemay
Endocrinology of Reproduction
Hospital Saint-Francoise D'Asise
Quebec G1L 3L5, Canada

David Levran
Interdepartmental Unit of Human Reproduction
Department of Obstetrics and Gynecology
The Chaim Sheba Medical Center and Sackler School of Medicine
Tel-Hashomer 52621, Israel

Joseph Levy
Endocrinology Laboratory, Soroka Medical Center and
Division of Obstetrics and Gynecology
Clinical Biochemistry Unit, Faculty of Health Sciences
Ben-Gurion University of the Negev
Beer-Sheba 84101, Israel

L. Levy
Tel Aviv University
Sackler School of Medicine
Tel Aviv, Israel

G. Leyendecker
Department of Obstetrics and Gynecology
Staedtische Kliniken, Grafenstrasse 9
D-6100 Darmstadt, FRG

D.F.H. Li
Department of Obstetrics and Gynecology
University of Hong Kong
Hong Kong

V. Lichtenburg
UKE Frauenklinik
Division of Endocrinology
Martinistrasse 52
2000 Hamburg 20, FRG

S.L. Lightman
Charing Cross and Westminster Medical School
London, UK

Ch. Lindner
UKE Frauenklinik
Division of Endocrinology
Martinistrasse 52
2000 Hamburg 20, FRG

Kathleen Link
Department of Medicine and Pediatrics
Harvard Medical School
Boston, MA 02115, USA

Schlomo Lipitz
Interdepartmental Unit of Human Reproduction
Department of Obstetrics and Gynecology
The Chaim Sheba Medical Center and Sackler School of Medicine
Tel-Hashomer 52621, Israel

A. Lipton
Department of Medicine/Endocrinology
Milton S. Hershey Medical Center
Pennsylvania State University
PO Box 850, Hershey, PA 17033, USA

P. Lopes
IVF Department
CHU Nantes
44035-Nantes Cedex 01, France

M. Luckhardt
UKE Frauenklinik
Division of Endocrinology
Martinistrasse 52
2000 Hamburg 20, FRG

Bruno Lunenfeld
Institute of Endocrinology
Sheba Medical Center and Bar Ilan University
Remat Gan 52621, Israel

E. Lunenfeld
Division of Obstetrics and Gynecology
Soroka Medical Center and Ben-Gurion University of the Negev
Beer-Sheba, Israel

J.L. McGuire
Ortho Pharmaceutical Corporation
Route 202
Raritan, NJ 08869, USA

Georgia I. McRae
Institute of Biological Sciences
Syntex Research
Palo Alto, CA 94304, USA

Gilles Manhes
Laval University Medical Center
Quebec G1V 4G2, Canada

Andrea Manni
Department of Medicine/Endocrinology
The Milton S. Hershey Medical Center
The Pennsylvania State University
PO Box 850, Hershey, PA 17033, USA

Joan Mansfield
Reproductive Endocrine Unit
Massachusetts General Hospital
Rear Blossom Street
Boston, MA 02114, USA

Shlomo Maschiach
Interdepartmental Unit of Human Reproduction
Department of Obstetrics and Gynecology
The Chaim Sheba Medical Center and Sackler School of Medicine
Tel-Hashomer 52621, Israel

W.H.M. Matta
Academic Department of Obstetrics and Gynaecology
Royal Free Hospital
London NW3 2QG, UK

Devorah T. Max
Abbott Laboratories
Abbott Park, IL 60064, USA

P. Merat
Pharmaceutical Division
Hoechst Canada Inc.
4045 Cote Vertu
Montreal, Quebec H4R 1R6, Canada

L. Mettler
Department of Obstetrics and Gynecology
University of Kiel
2300 Kiel, FRG

E. Milliet
Gynecologie-Obstetrique
Hopital Michael Levy, Annexe Conception
84a rue de Lodi
13281 Marseille Cedex 6, France

H.W. Minne
Department of Internal Medicine
University of Heidelberg
Heidelberg, FRG

Gerard Monfette
Laval University Medical Center
Quebec G1V 4G2, Canada

A. Morini
First Institute of Obstetrics and Gynecology
University "La Sapienza"
Rome, Italy

H. Nachum
Department of Obstetrics and Gynecology
Assaf Harofe Medical Center
Zerefin, Israel

John J. Nestor Jr.
Institute of Bio-Organic Chemistry
Syntex Research
3401 Hillview Avenue
Palo Alto, CA 94304, USA

J. Neulen
Department of Obstetrics and Gynecology
Division of Clinical Endocrinology
University of Freiburg
D-7800 Freiburg-im-Breisgau, FRG

D. Newling
A.Z. Middelheim
Antwerp 2020, Belgium

Eberhard Nieschlag
Max Planck Clinical Research Unit for Reproductive Medicine
Institute of Reproductive Medicine of the University
D-4400 Münster, FRG

F. Oberheuser
Klinik für Franenheilkunde und Geburtshilfe
Institute für Biochemische Endokrinologie
Medizinische Universiteit zu Lübeck
D-2400 Lübeck, FRG

A.J.H. Odink
Sophia Children's Hospital
160 Gordelweg
3038 GE Rotterdam, The Netherlands

E.P.N. O'Donohue
Department of Urology
Central Middlesex Hospital
London, UK

P. Onegana
A.Z. Middelheim
Antwerp 2020, Belgium

W. Oostdijk
Sophia Children's Hospital
160 Gordelweg
3038 GE Rotterdam, The Netherlands

G.S. Pahwa
Klinik für Franenheilkunde und Gerburtshilfe
Institute für Biochemische Endokrinologie
Medizinische Universiteit zu Lübeck
D-2400 Lübeck, FRG

Christopher A. Palabrica
Pharmaceutical Discovery Division
Abbott Laboratories
Abbott Park, IL 60064, USA

I. Papadopoulos
Urologische Universitatsklinik Kiel
Arnold-Heller Strasse 7
D-2300 Kiel 1, FRG

H. Parmar
Department of Oncology
Westminster Hospital
London SW1 2AP, UK

C.J. Partsch
Sophia Children's Hospital
160 Gordelweg
3038 GE Rotterdam, The Netherlands

Spyros N. Pavlou
Division of Endocrinology
Vanderbilt University School of Medicine
Nashville, TN 37232, USA

Peg Pepping
Section of Reproductive
Endocrinology/Infertility
Department of Obstetrics and Gynecology
Rush Medical Center
Chicago, IL 60612, USA

A. Phillips
Ortho Pharmaceutical Corporation
Route 202
Raritan, NJ 08869, USA

R.H. Phillips
Westminster Hospital
London SW1 2AP, UK

F. Piccinno
First Institute of Obstetrics and
Gynecology
University "La Sapienza"
Rome, Italy

G. Potashnik
Division of Obstetrics and Gynecology
Soroka Medical Center and Ben Gurion
University of the Negev
Beer Sheba, Israel

P. Puttemans
Laboratory for Gynaecological
Pathophysiology
Gasthuisberg
KU Leuven, Belgium

Ewa Radwanska
Section of Reproductive
Endocrinology/Infertility
Department of Obstetrics and Gynecology
Rush Medical College
Chicago, IL 60612, USA

R. Rappaport
Unit of Pediatric Endocrinology and
Diabetes
Hospital des Enfants Malades
75015 Paris, France

Tommie W. Redding
Veterans Administration Medical Center
1601 Perdido Street
New Orleans, LA 71046, USA

D.M. Ritchie
Ortho Pharmaceutical Corporation
Route 202
Raritan, NJ 08869, USA

Jean Rivier
Salk Institute for Biological Studies
La Jolla, CA 92037, USA

A. Rodin
Department of Gynaecology
Guy's Hospital
London, UK

M. Roger
Foundation de Recherche en
Hormonologie
PB110
94268 Fresnes Cedex, France

T. Rohner
Department of Medicine/Endocrinology
Milton S. Hershey Medical Center
Pennsylvania State University
PO Box 850, Hershey, PA 17033, USA

R. Ron-El
Department of Obstetrics and Gynecology
Assaf Harofe Medical Center
Zerefin, Israel

Edwina Rudak
Interdepartmental Unit of Human
Reproduction
Department of Obstetrics and Gynecology
The Chaim Sheba Medical Center and
Sackler School of Medicine
Tel-Hashomer 52621, Israel

Benno Runnebaum
Division of Gynecological Endocrinology
Department of Obstetrics and Gynecology
University of Heidelberg
D-6900 Heidelberg, FRG

D. Sala
First Institute of Obstetrics and Gynecology
Rome, Italy

Lynda M. Sanders
Institute of Pharmaceutical Sciences
Syntex Research
Palo Alto, CA 94304, USA

Jurgen Sandow
Department of Pharmacology
Hoechst AG
D-6230 Frankfurt 80, FRG

R. Santen
Department of Medicine/Endocrinology
Milton S. Hershey Medical Center
Pennsylvania State University
PO Box 850, Hershey, PA 17033, USA

Carlos A. Schaffenburg
5480 Wisconsin Avenue 1014
Chevy Chase, MD 20815, USA

Andrew V. Schally
Endocrine Polypeptide and Cancer Institute
Veterans Admininstration Medical Center and Section of Experimental Medicine
Department of Medicine, Tulane University School of Medicine
New Orleans, LA 70146, USA

S.H. Scharla
Department of Internal Medicine
University of Heidelberg
Heidelberg, FRG

F. Schaumkell
Urologische Universitatsklinik Kiel
Arnold-Heller Strasse 7
D-2300 Kiel 1, FRG

H. Schillinger
Department of Obstetrics and Gynecology
Division of Clinical Endocrinology
University of Freiburg
D-7800 Freiburg-im-Breisgau, FRG

T. Schlotfeld
UKE Frauenklinik
Division of Endocrinology
Martinistrasse 52
2000 Hamburg 20, FRG

R. Scholler
Foundation de Recherche en Hormonologie
PB110
94268 Fresnes Cedex, France

John H. Seely
Abbott Laboratories
Abbott Park, IL 60064, USA

Tzuria Segal
Endocrinology Laboratory, Soroka Medical Center and
Division of Obstetrics and Gynecology
Clinical Biochemistry Unit, Faculty of Health Sciences
Ben Gurion University of the Negev
Beer-Sheba 84101, Israel

Yoav Sharoni
Endocrinology Laboratory, Soroka Medical Center and
Division of Obstetrics and Gynecology
Clinical Biochemistry Unit, Faculty of Health Sciences
Ben Gurion University of the Negev
Beer-Sheba 84101, Israel

R.W. Shaw
Academic Department of Obstetrics and Gynecology
Royal Free Hospital School of Medicine
London NW3, UK

R. Shiffl
Department of Internal Medicine
University of Heidelberg
Heidelberg, FRG

Karol Sikora
Department of Clinical Oncology
Hammersmith Hospital
DuCane Road
London W12 OHS, UK

M. Simmonds
Department of Medicine/Endocrinology
Milton S. Hershey Medical Center
Pennsylvania State University
PO Box 850, Hershey, PA 17033, USA

W.G. Sippell
Sophia Children's Hospital
160 Goodelweg
3038 GE Rotterdam, The Netherlands

Pierre C. Sizonenko
Department of Pediatrics and Genetics
Division of Biology of Growth and Reproduction
University of Geneva Medical School
1211 Geneva 4, Switzerland

P.H. Smith
A.Z. Middelheim
Antwerp 2020, Belgium

J. Smitz
Center for Reproductive Medicine
Medical Campus, Vrije Universiteit Brussel
Laarbeeklaan 101
1090 Brussels, Belgium

Y. Soffer
Department of Obstetrics and Gynecology
Assaf Harofe Medical Center
Zerefin, Israel

C. Staesson
Center for Reproductive Medicine
Medical Campus, Vrije Universiteit Brussel
Laarbeeklaan 101
1090 Brussels, Belgium

David Stephure
Department of Pediatrics
University of California San Francisco
San Francisco, CA 94943, USA

R. Strum
Klinik für Franenheilkunde und Geburtshilfe
Institut für Biochemische Endokrinologie
Medizinische Universiteit zu Lübeck
D-2400 Lübeck, FRG

Linda J. Swanson
Abbott Laboratories
Abbott Park, IL 60064, USA

R. Sylvester
A.Z. Middelheim
Antwerp 2020, Belgium

G.P. Taylor
Departments of Pediatrics and Pathology
University of British Columbia
BC's Children's Hospital
Vancouver, BC V6H 3V4, Canada

J.E. Toublanc
Foundation de Recherche en Hormonologie
PB110
94268 Fresnes Cedex, France

Ian Tummon
Section of Reproductive Endocrinology/Infertility
Department of Obstetrics and Gynecology
Rush Medical College
Chicago, IL 60612, USA

W.J. Tze
Department of Pediatrics and Pathology
University of British Columbia
BC's Children's Hospital
Vancouver, BC V6H 3V4, Canada

Wylie Vale
Salk Institute for Biological Studies
La Jolla, CA 92037, USA

A.N. van Geel
Department of Surgery
The Rotterdam Cancer Institute
Rotterdam, The Netherlands

A.C. Van Steirteghen
Center for Reproductive Medicine
Medical Campus, Vrije Universiteit Brussel
Laarbeeklaan 101
1090 Brussels, Belgium

L. Van Waesberghe
Center for Reproductive Medicine
Medical Campus, Vrije Universiteit Brussel
Laarbeeklaan 101
1090 Brussels, Belgium

Brian H. Vickery
Institute of Biological Sciences
Syntex Research
Palo Alto, CA 94304, USA

W. von Rechenberg
Hoechst AG
D-6230 Frankfurt 80, FRG

S. Waibel
Department of Obstetrics and Gynecology
Staedtische Kliniken
Grafenstrasse 9
D-6100 Darmstadt, FRG

H. Wand
Urologische Universitatsklinik Kiel
Arnold-Heller Strasse 7
D-2300 Kiel 1, FRG

Jonathan Waxman
Department of Clinical Oncology
Hammersmith Hospital
DuCane Road
London W12 OHS, UK

Gerhard F. Weinbauer
Max Planck Clinical Research Unit for Reproductive Medicine
Institute of Reproductive Medicine of the University
D-4400 Münster, FRG

Z. Weinraub
Department of Obstetrics and Gynecology
Assaf Hasofe Medical Center
Zerefin, Israel

J. Wettlaufer
Department of Medicine/Endocrinology
Milton S. Hershey Medical Center
Pennsylvania State University
PO Box 850, Hershey, PA 17033, USA

D. White-Hershey
Department of Medicine/Endocrinology
Milton S. Hershey Medical Center
Pennsylvania State University
PO Box 850, Hershey, PA 17033, USA

L. Wildt
Department of Gynecology and Obstetrics
University of Erlangen-Nürnberg
8520 Erlangen, FRG

G. Williams
Department of Urology
Hammersmith Hospital
DuCane Road
London W12 OHS, UK

A. Wisanto
Center for Reproductive Medicine
Medical Campus, Vrije Universiteit Brussel
Laarbeeklaan 101
1090 Brussels, Belgium

Arnon Wiznitzer
Endocrinology Laboratory, Soroka Medical Center and
Division of Obstetrics and Gynecology
Clinical Biochemistry Unit, Faculty of Health Sciences
Ben-Gurion University of the Negev
Beer-Sheba 84101, Israel

C. Wüster
Department of Internal Medicine
University of Heidelberg
Heidelberg, FRG

Attila Zalatnai
Veterans Administration Medical Center
1601 Perdido Street
New Orleans, LA 71046, USA

R. Ziegler
Department of Internal Medicine
University of Heidelberg
Heidelberg, FRG

1

IS THERE A RATIONALE FOR GnRH ANALOGUE THERAPY IN ENDOMETRIOSIS?

Ivo A. BROSENS, Freddy CORNILLIE and **Patrick PUTTEMANS**
Laboratory of Gynaecological Physiopathology,
University Hospital Gasthuisberg, Catholic University of Leuven (KUL),
Leuven, Belgium
and Department of Obstetrics and Gynaecology,
KUL - UCL Hospital St. Elisabeth, Brussels, Belgium

INTRODUCTION

Although endometriosis is considered as the most common benign gynaecological disease in women during their reproductive years and despite many hundreds of articles having been written on the subject, much controversy remains regarding its pathogenesis, pathophysiology and therapy. In this paper the criteria for diagnosis and evaluation of response to medical therapy will be discussed.

CLINICAL APPEARANCE AND DIAGNOSIS

More than 60 years ago Sampson described in great detail the various appearances of endometriosis [1-3]. He carefully observed different types of endometriosis such as the red, dark brown and black lesions embedded in fibrotic tissue as well as oedematous vesiculi. Although these observations were well documented, the nodular thickening noted on palpation of the posterior cul-de-sac and utero-sacral ligaments has been the outstanding finding on vaginal and rectal examination for the diagnosis of endometriosis. The characteristic appearance of ectopic implants was that of blueberry-like spots surrounded by a puckering scar. These nodules represent the most readily recognizable stigmata of disease at laparoscopy or laparotomy. This has led some authors to conclude that endometriosis can be accurately diagnosed by inspection.

More recently, several authors [4-7] have drawn attention to the variety of appearances of peritoneal endometriosis. In addition, microscopic peritoneal endometriosis has been described [8-9]. The implications on the pathophysiology of these different implants of endometriosis are not clear, but evidence is emerging that these implants may have a different effect on the constituents of peritoneal fluid [10].

Three types of peritoneal implants of endometriosis can be distinguished:

1 **Endometrial vesicles** have a diameter of 1 to 3 mm and are usually haemorrhagic. In the absence of bleeding the colour is clear or straw-yellow. By contact laparoscopy the fine vascular network can be seen. On histology these implants represent active, frequently cystic or polypoid endometrial tissue covered by mesothelium. The implants are highly vascularized and the glandular epithelium manifests the cyclic changes of the menstrual cycle [11]. The non-haemorrhagic type of vesicle or papule has to be differentiated by histology from other peritoneal lesions such as vesicular inflammatory or infectious lesions, foreign body reactions or fibrin deposits. On the other hand, subperitoneal dilated venules and capillaries may also represent false positives and mimic hamorrhagic implants of endometriosis [12].

2. The **nodular lesions** represent a different type of implant of endometriosis. The colour can vary from white, yellow or red to brown or black. On histological examination endometrial tissue is found in approximately 50% of the biopsies. Deposits of hemosiderin are frequently found in these lesions and are related to the colour of the implant [10]. The implant is poorly vascularized and epithelial activity is usually absent. Fibrosis and a puckering scar seem to be intent on drawing other tissue into the lesion.

3. The **epithelial plaque-type implant** is an area of columnar or cuboidal surface epithelium in continuity with the mesothelial lining of the peritoneal cavity. This lesion is usually well differentiated and active but is not easily detected at laparoscopy. The endometrial epithelium is in direct contact with the peritoneal cavity and therefore this lesion can be considered as intraperitoneal endometriosis.

Endometrial ovarian cysts also can have different appearances and represent a major diagnostic problem. The term "chocolate cyst" of the ovary is descriptive and it lends itself readily to misinterpretation if one notices only the chocolate-coloured haemorrhagic content. A somewhat similar content may be found in some follicle or lutein haematomas or even in a cystic adenoma.

Recent endoscopic exploration of endometrial ovarian cysts has revealed that the wall of the cyst is poorly vascularized and that sinusoidal veins protrude on the surface in the area of the hilus of the ovary. Histologically the wall of the cyst is largely composed of fibrotic tissue with poor vascularization and a variable amount of endometrial elements. The endometrial glands tend to be cystic or atrophic and show little evidence of cyclic hormonal changes during the menstrual cycle. It is possible that the haemorrhagic content of the endometrial ovarian cyst is derived from chronic bleeding of the congested veins in the hilus of the ovary rather than from endometrial shedding at the time of menstruation. Peritoneal implants are frequently sited at the hilus of the ovary in the fossa ovarica. The associated inflammatory reaction, fibrosis and retraction may cause venous congestion and chronic bleeding and lead to the formation of a unilocular haemorrhagic cyst adherent to the fossa ovarica.

HORMONAL MODULATION

Studies comparing the ectopic and eutopic endometrium have shown that, although the ectopic implant can be assigned to a particular phase of the cycle, the response to the prevalent milieu is usually incomplete or inadequate. Ultrastructural studies have shown that full secretory transformation with the development of the so-called postovulatory functional triad (i.e. giant mitochondria, nuclear channel system and glycogen accumulation) is absent in ectopic endometrium. The inadequate cyclical changes of endometriotic implants are related to the low concentrations of steroid receptors found in these lesions. It was suggested by Jånne and colleagues [13] that there is a higher incidence of progesterone receptors in mild disease than in severe or extensive lesions. A very low number of cytoplasmic oestrogen receptors have been found in ovarian endometriosis. The wide variations of histologic and cytologic appearance within endometriotic lesions as well as their differences from the eutopic endometrium may relate to the completely different vascular supply [12]. A good microvascular supply is a prerequisite for the normal and hormonally modulated synthesis of steroid receptors within ectopic endometrium.

RESPONSE TO THERAPY

Laparoscopic evaluation

Clinical studies of the medical therapy of endometriosis are faced with major difficulties in evaluating the effect of treatment. Laparoscopy is usually performed before and at the end of therapy and stages of endometriosis are scored. Various degrees of resolution have been described at the end of a long-term therapy [14]. However, observations before and at the end of medical therapy usually compare the appearances of the implant under different hormonal conditions, i.e. during cyclic versus suppressed ovarian activity. The basic question, however, is whether medical therapy has an effect on the implant in terms of tissue degeneration and cell loss. Prolonged inactivation results in resorption of the manifestations of activity such as vesicle formation and haemorrhage but not necessarily in cell loss. A so-called "clean" pelvis at the end of longterm hormonal therapy involving suppression of ovarian activity is no proof that the implants have resolved.

The transient effect of medical therapy on the enhancement of fertility and the high recurrence rate suggest that the beneficial effect of hormonal therapy of endometriosis results from a temporary inactivation of the implant rather than from eradication of the disease. Inactivation of the implant can probably be achieved by a shorter therapy than necessary for full resorption [15]. The question therefore remains whether medical therapy of pelvic endometriosis to enhance fertility benefits substantially from prolongation.

Morphological response to hormonal therapy

Studies of the effect of danazol, Gestrinone and GnRH agonists on endometriotic tissue has shown that these products induce cellular inactivity and degeneration [11, 12, 16]. Two types of cellular involution have been described. The first type is characterized by an increased number of lysosomes and autophagic vacuoles as well as nuclear changes and pycnosis. Endometriotic epithelial cells with this type of cytoplasmic and nuclear involution become necrotic and are shed from the basement membrane. However, the common finding is cytoplasmic disintegration due to enhanced lysosomal activity while nuclear degenerative changes occur only in a minority of cells. Another type of cellular change is characterized by cytoplasmic lipid overload without obvious cellular degeneration. This second type of change has been seen after danazol therapy (600mg daily) but not after Gestrinone therapy (2.5mg twice or thrice weekly) or GnRH agonists. Since only the first type of involution results in pycnosis, cellular fragmentation and extrusion of cell nuclei, it may be concluded that only this type of cellular degeneration can eliminate individual endometriotic epithelial cells and resolve the implant. Shorter two-month therapy with a higher dose of Gestrinone can inactivate all implants (Table 1). These data support the hypothesis that the derivatives of 17α-ethinyl testosterone induce a progesterone withdrawal effect at the

TABLE 1: Effect of 2- and 4-months therapy in peritoneal endometriosis.

Implant	4 months Gestrinone (2.5 mg 2-3 x weekly)	2 months Gestrinone (1.25 mg daily)
Active	6 (42%)	0 (0%)
At rest	4 (29%)	9 (56%)
Involuntary	4 (29%)	7 (44%)

cellular level resulting in enhanced lysosomal degradation of epithelial cells.

The most significant difference between pre- and post treatment morphology in patients treated with GnRH agonists is the increase of involutionary implants (Table 2). However, after three-months therapy with intranasal buserelin 300μg tid, 17% of the implants were still active. Further morphological studies are in progress to evaluate the effect of longer duration of therapy and other routes of administration of GnRH agonists.

TABLE 2: Effect of Buserelin intranasal spray on peritoneal implants of endometriosis after 3 months of therapy.

Implant	Before therapy	After therapy
Active	5 (42%)	2 (17%)
At rest	6 (50%)	3 (25%)
Involuntary	1 (8%)	7 (58%)

CONCLUSIONS

Minimal or mild endometriosis (as defined by the AFS classification system) is not a homogeneous disease in terms of amount or activity of ectopic endometrial tissue. Three different types of peritoneal implants can be distinguished: the active, vesicular implant; the inactive fibrotic and pigmented implant; and the active intraperitoneal surface implant. The last type is microscopic and is not observed at laparoscopy.

The effect of medical therapy on endometriotic implants is not accurately reflected by their appearance at laparoscopy. To evaluate the effect of medical treatment by laparoscopy alone, the observations should be performed under similar endocrine condiions. Biopsies provide a more accurate evaluation of the effect of medical therapy.

Buserelin intranasal spray therapy at the level of 300μg tid produces involutionary changes in the majority of implants after 3 months. However, the effect is variable as 17% of the implants still remain active at this time.

REFERENCES

1. Sampson, JA (1921). Perforating hemorrhagic (chocolate) cysts of the ovary, their importance and especially their relation of pelvic adenomas of the endometrial type. Arch Surg, 3, 245
2. Sampson, JA (1924). Benign and malignant implants in the peritoneal cavity and their relation to certain ovarian tumors. Surg Gynecol Obstet, 32, 287
3. Sampson, JA (1927). Peritoneal endometriosis due to menstrual dissemination of endometrial tissue into the peritoneal cavity. Am J Obstet Gynecol, 14, 422
4. Chatman, DL (1981). Pelvic peritoneal defects and endometriosis: Allen-Masters syndrome revisited. Fertil Steril, 36, 751
5. Chatman, DL and Zbella, EA (1986). Pelvic peritoneal defects and endometriosis: further observations. Fertil Steril, 47, 711
6. Redwine, DBA (1985). Atypical endometriosis. In Prog Ann Meet Am Fert Soc, 64 (Abstract)
7. Jansen, RPS and Russell, P (1986). Nonpigmented endometriosis: clinical, laparoscopic and pathologic definition. Am J Obstet Gynecol, 155, 1154
8. Vasquez, G, Cornillie, F and Brosens, IA (1984). Peritoneal endometriosis: scanning electron microscopy and histology of minimal pelvic endometriotic lesions. Fertil Steril, 42, 496
9. Murphy, AA, Green, WR, Bobbie, D, dela Cruz, ZC and Rock, JA (1987). Unsuspected endometriosis documented by scanning electron microscopy in visually normal peritoneum. Fertil Steril, 46, 522
10. Vernon, MW, Beard, JS, Graves, K and Wilson, EA (1986). Classification of endometriotic implants by morphologic appearance and capacity to synthesize prostaglandin. Fertil Steril, 46, 801
11. Cornillie, FJ, Brosens, IA, Vasquez, G and Riphagen, I (1986). Histologic and ultrastructural changes in human endometriotic implants treated with antiprogesterone steroid ethylnorgestrinone (gestrinone) during 2 months. Int J Gynecol Path, 5, 95
12. Brosens, IA, Cornillie, FJ and Fasquez, G (1986). Etiology and pathophysiology of endometriosis. In: Rolland, R, Chadha Dev, R, Willemsen, WNP (eds.) "Gonadotrophin Down-Regulation in Gynecological Practice". Vol 81, p.102. (New York: Alan R. Liss)
13. Jânne, O, Kauppila, A, Kokko, E, Lanto, T, Ronnberg, L and Vikko, R (1981). Estrogen and progestin receptors in endometriosis lesions: Comparison with endometrial tissue. Am J Obstet Gynecol, 141, 562
14. Buttram, VC Jr (1985). Treatment of endometriosis with danazol: report of a 6-year prospective study. Fertil Steril, 43, 353
15. Brosens, IA, Verleyen, A and Cornillie, F (1987). The morphologic effect of short-term medical therapy of endometriosis. Am J Obstet Gynecol, 157, 1215
16. Schweppe, KW, Dmowski, WP and Wynn, RM (1981). Ultrastructural changes in endometriotic tissue during danazal treatment. Fertil Steril, 36, 20

2

GnRH AGONISTS IN THE MANAGEMENT OF ENDOMETRIOSIS: THE RESULTS OF TWO RANDOMIZED TRIALS

W. Paul DMOWSKI, Ewa RADWANSKA, Zvi BINOR, Ian TUMMON and **Peg PEPPING**
Section of Reproductive Endocrinology/Infertility,
Department of Obstetrics and Gynecology Rush Medical College,
Chicago, Illinois 60612, USA

INTRODUCTION

Endometriosis is a perplexing disease of unknown etiology and poorly understood histogenesis. It affects women as well as menstruating females of other primate species and is characterized by ectopic i.e., outside of the uterine cavity, growth of endometrium. The growth and spread of endometriosis are controlled by the cyclic stimulation of ovarian hormones. After cessation of ovarian function e.g., during menopause, when ovarian estradiol and progesterone are no longer secreted, uterine as well as ectopic endometria undergo atrophy and endometriosis resolves.

For this reason, temporary suppression of ovarian function is the principle of hormonal treatment in endometriosis. For more than a decade danazol-induced "pseudomenopause" has been the main hormonal approach in the management of endometriosis and endometriosis-related infertility [1]. Symptomatic and clinical improvement and regression of endometriotic lesions during pseudomenopause have been generally considered as satisfactory and are typically followed by post-treatment improvement in fertility. However, the disease often returns when menstrual cycles are reestablished and danazol, a steroid with androgenic properties, displays a variety of side effects, which some patients find difficult to accept.

Gonadotropin releasing hormone agonists (GnRH-a) are structural analogues to native GnRH. Administered parenterally they initially stimulate gonadotropin release but with continuous administration of the agonist, pituitary receptors are downregulated and FSH and LH release is inhibited. Consequently, after about two weeks of treatment ovarian function is also suppressed. The degree of ovarian suppression during GnRH-a administration is greater than that achieved with danazol [2]. Recently several GnRH agonists have been found effective in the clinical management of endometriosis and resolution of endometriotic lesions has been observed during preliminary clinical trials with these compounds [2].

The purpose of this study was to compare the effectiveness of two GnRH agonists with that of danazol in the management of endometriosis.

MATERIALS AND METHODS

Fifty-one women of child-bearing age with laparoscopically diagnosed and staged endometriosis [3] were enrolled in two open label prospective clinical trials. In the first study 36 patients were enrolled and were randomized to buserelin intranasal (IN) 0.4mg TID, buserelin subcutaneous (SC) 0.2mg daily or to danazol 800mg daily. Twenty-nine patients completed the study; of those 10 received buserelin IN, 9 buserelin SC, and 10 danazol. In the second study, 15 patients were enrolled and all completed the study. They were randomized to leuprolide 0.5mg SC daily for one week, then 0.4mg IN QID (10) or to danazol 800mg daily (5). The treatment with buserelin, leuprolide or danazol was continued for six months, when repeat laparoscopic assessment was performed. Symptomatic, clinical and hormonal evaluations were performed at monthly intervals in all patients. Pelvic pain scores, consisting of a total score for dysmenorrhea, dyspareunia and pelvic pain on the 0-3 point scale in a buserelin study and 1-10 point analog scale in the leuprolide study, were recorded at each visit. Patients with ovarian endometriomas larger than 3cm had serial pelvic ultrasonograms before, during and after treatment. Bone mineral density (BMD) measurements were performed, with dual photon absorptiometry (DPA) of the lumbar spine, before and after treatment. The results were reported as percent of the mean of control population from the same geographical region matched for race, age and weight. On the last day of treatment repeat laparoscopy was performed and again the extent of endometriosis was evaluated according to the American Fertility Society scoring system [3]. Side effects of treatment and their intensity were recorded on a 0-3 point scale during each visit. Only side effects reported at two consecutive visits four weeks apart were considered in the final analysis. Cumulative pregnancy rates were calculated for both groups during the 12-month post treatment follow-up period [4].

RESULTS

During treatment, amenorrhea and suppressed FSH, LH, estradiol and progesterone levels were observed in all patients (Tables 1 and 2). In the buserelin study there were no significant differences in mean cumulative estradiol, FSH or LH levels between buserelin IN, SC or danazol treated patients. However, mean estradiol levels at week 16 were higher in danazol than buserelin groups ($P<0.05$) and mean LH levels were higher at week 8 in buserelin SC than in other groups ($P<0.05$). Mean cumulative progesterone levels were higher in danazol than buserelin groups (Table 1). In the leuprolide study mean cumulative estradiol and progesterone levels were significantly higher in the danazol group. Although there were no significant differences in mean cumulative FSH and LH levels between the groups in that study, both FSH and LH levels were higher at weeks 4, 8 and 12 in the danazol group ($P<0.05$).

TABLE 1: Endocrine changes during ovarian suppression with buserelin or danazol.

Group	N	E_2 (pg/ml)	FSH (mIU/ml)	LH (mIU/ml)	P (ng/ml)
buserelin (1.2mg IN)	10	36 ± 5*	10 ± 0.5	10 ± 0.6	0.3 ± 0.03
buserelin (0.2mg SC)	9	33 ± 2	11 ± 0.4	13 ± 0.5	0.3 ± 0.01
danazol (800mg)	10	39 ± 4	11 ± 0.4	10 ± 0.5	0.4 ± 0.02
significance		NS	NS	NS	$p<0.05$

*mean ± SEM

TABLE 2: Endocrine changes during ovarian suppression with leuprolide or danazol.

Group	N	E_2 (pg/ml)	FSH (mIU/ml)	LH (mIU/ml)	P (ng/ml)
leuprolide (1.6mg IN)	10	23 ± 2*	9 ± 0.1	9 ± 0.9	0.2 ± 0.01
danazol (800mg)	5	41 ± 4	12 ± 0.3	12 ± 0.7	0.4 ± 0.01
significance		$p<0.01$	NS	NS	$p<0.01$

*mean ± SEM

Symptomatic improvement, simultaneous with the development of amenorrhea, was recorded in all patients and pelvic pain scores decreased significantly during treatment (Tables 3 and 4). The size of ovarian endometriomas larger than 3cm decreased by an average of 40% in GnRH-a treated and by 47% in danazol treated

TABLE 3: Pelvic pain scores* before and at the end of treatment with buserelin or danazol.

Group	N	Pretreatment	Post treatment	Significance
buserelin (IN or SC)	19	2.7 ± 0.5**	0.7 ± 0.2	$p<0.02$
danazol (800mg)	10	3.3 ± 0.5	0.4 ± 0.2	$p<0.02$

*Total dysmenorrhea, dyspareunia and pelvic pain scores on a 0-3 point scale.
**Mean ± SEM

TABLE 4: Pelvic pain scores* before and at the end of treatment with leuprolide or danazol.

Group	N	Pretreatment	Post treatment	Significance
leuprolise (1.6mg IN)	10	3.0 ± 0.6**	0.4 ± 0.2	$p<0.05$
danazol (800mg)	5	3.4 ± 2.0	1.4 ± 0.7	$p<0.05$

*Total dysmenorrhea, dyspareunia and pelvic pain scores on a 1-10 point scale.
**Mean ± SEM

patients (P=NS). BMD measurements before and after treatment with GnRH-a or danazol are given in Table 5. There were no significant changes in BMD during ovarian suppression with either regimen. Repeat laparoscopy demonstrated a significant decrease in the extent of endometriosis in all patients. The revised American Fertility Society scores for endometriosis before and after treatment are given in Tables 6 and 7. During 12

TABLE 5: Bone mineral density (BMD)* before and after 26 weeks of ovarian suppression withGnRH-a or danazol.

Group	N	Before	After	Significance
GnRH-a	21	98.9 ± 0.5**	98.6 ± 0.02	NS
danazol	12	95.3 ± 0.8	95.8 ± 2.7	NS

*% of control population matched for race, age and weight
**Mean ± SEM

TABLE 6: Endometriosis scores at laparoscopy* before and after treatment buserelin or danazol.

	N	Before	After	Chance	Significanc
buserelin (1.2mg IN)	10	28 ± 7**	18 ± 7	10 ± 4	p<0.02
buserelin (0.2mg SC)	9	27 ± 7	9 ± 3	18 ± 6	p<0.02
danazol (800mg)	10	20 ± 4	7 ± 3	13 ± 3	p<0.02

*Revised American Fertility Society Classification
**Men ± SEM

months of follow-up, conception occurred in 7 of 10 infertile women treated with leuprolide (70%), in 7 of 17 treated with buserelin (47%) and in 7 of 13 treated with danazol (54%). The cumulative pregnancy rates after treatment with GnRH-a or danazol are given in Figure 1.

One or more side effects of treatment were reported by all patients treated with buserelin, leuprolide or danazol. However, the frequency and intensity of side effects varied. They were similar in two GnRH-a groups and different in the danazol group (Table 8). Vasomotor side effects were more pronounced in the

TABLE 7: Endometriosis scores at laparoscopy* before and after treatment leuprolide or danazol.

Group	N	Before	After	Chance	Significance
leuprolise (1.6mg IN)	10	24 ± 7**	11 ± 5	13 ± 3	$p<0.05$
danazol (800mg)	5	18 ± 4	5 ± 3	13 ± 4	$p<0.05$

*Revised American Fertility Society Classification
*Mean ± SEM

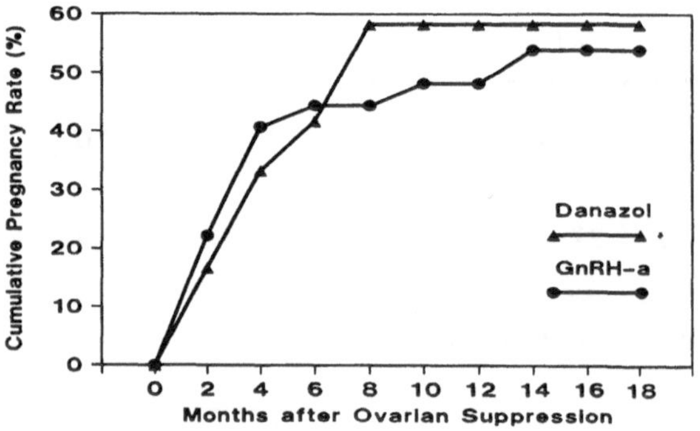

FIGURE 1 Cumulative pregnancy rates after ovarian suppression with GnRH-a or danazol

GnRH-a groups especially during the last eight weeks of treatment. However, the difference between GnRH-a and danazol treatment patients was not significant. There were no significant differences in the intensity of vaginal dryness, headaches, sleep disturbances, irritability, depression or fatigue between GnRH-a and danazol groups. Acne and oily skin was observed more

TABLE 8: Frequency of side effects during ovarian suppression with GnRH-a or danazol.

Side effect	GnRH-A (%)	Danazol (%)	Significance
vasomotor symptoms	86	60	NS
vaginal dryness	45	27	NS
sleep disturbances	14	27	NS
headaches	38	27	NS
irritability	28	40	NS
depression	17	27	NS
fatigue	28	27	NS
acne/oily skin	17	53	$p<0.05$
weight gain > 5 lbs	21	60	$p<0.05$

frequently in the danazol group and the intensity of these changes was higher. Weight gain of more than 5 pounds was more frequent in the danazol group. Hirsutism, voice changes and other frank androgenic side effects were not observed. Seven patients in the buserelin study did not complete the protocol. Three were in the SC group, two in IN and two in danazol. There were no consistent reasons for discontinuation of the study. Two patients reported family reasons, three were non-compliant, one had severe emotional side effects on IN buserelin and one was allergic to danazol.

CONCLUSIONS

The results of our studies indicate that danazol and GnRH-a are capable of inducing a comparable degree of ovarian suppression in women with endometriosis. There was no significant difference in the cumulative mean estradiol, FSH and LH levels during treatment with 800mg/day of danazol, or buserelin administration IN or SC. It should be kept in mind, however, that at 800mg/day of danazol the maximum antigonadotropin effect has already been reached [1]. This may not be the case for buserelin which, at a dose higher than that used in our study, induced a more profound suppression of FSH, LH and estradiol [5]. Certainly, leuprolide in a higher IN dose, which followed a week long SC administration, had a more pronounced suppressive effect on the pituitary function. Mean estradiol levels were significantly lower in the leuprolide than in the danazol group and FSH and LH declines reached levels bordering on statistical significance. Interestingly, serum progesterone levels were consistently higher in danazol than in buserelin or leuprolide treated patients. This finding probably reflects an inhibitory effect of danazol on adrenal steroidogenesis. A similar finding was observed during treatment of ovariectomized rats with danazol but not with GnRH-a [6].

The degree of symptomatic and clinical improvement was comparable in all groups and there were no differences in this respect between danazol and either of the two GnRH-a regimens. The resolution of endometriosis, as judged by laparoscopic evaluation, was also similar with both regimens. Large endometriomas decreased in size during ovarian suppression with either danazol or GnRH-a, facilitating microsurgical resection at the end of the medical therapy. Contrary to earlier reports [7, 8], we found no significant changes in BMD during GnRH-a treatment. The fertility of infertile women improved and there was no difference in cumulative pregnancy rates after treatment with GnRH-a or danazol. The frequency of side effects related to the hypoestrogenic state was similar in GnRH-a and in danazol treated patients. However, mild androgenic and anabolic side effects were more frequent in the danazol group.

We conclude that GnRH agonists are comparable to danazol in their ability to suppress ovarian function and endometriosis and that they have fewer androgenic and anabolic side effects. They offer an attractive alternative to danazol in the medical management of endometriosis.

REFERENCES

1. Dmowski, WP (1988). Danazol induced pseudomenopause in the management of endometriosis. In R. Rebar (ed.) Clinical Obstetrics and Gynecology, in press
2. Meldrum, DR (1985). Clinical management of endometriosis with luteinizing hormone-releasing hormone analogues. Semin Reprod Endocrinol, 3, 371
3. The American Fertility Society (1985). Revised American fertility society classification of endometriosis. Fertil Steril, 43, 351
4. Lee, E (1980). "Statistical Methods for Survival Data Analysis." (Wadsworth, Belmont)
5. Lemay, A, Maheux, R, Faure, N, Jean, C, and Fazekas, ATA (1984). Reversible hypogonadism induced by a luteinizing hormone-releasing hormone (LH-RH) agonist (Buserelin) as a new therapeutic approach for endometriosis. Fertil Steril, 41, 863
6. Henig, I, Rawlins, RG, Weinrib, HP and Dmowski, WP (1988). Effects of danazol, gonadotropin releasing hormone agonist and

estrogen/progestogen combination on experimental endometriosis in the ovariectomized rat. Fertil Steril, in press
7. Cann, CE, Henzl, M, Burry, K, Andreko, J, Hanson, F, Adamson, D and Trobough, G (1986). Reversible bone loss is induced by GnRH agonists. Program of the Endocrine Society 68th Annual Meeting, June 25-27, Anaheim, CA
8. Lewis, V, Ramos, J, and Dawood, MY (1987). Changes in bone mineral content in endometriosis patients treated with GnRH agonist. Program of the Society for Gynecologic Investigation 34th Annual Meeting, March 18-21, Atlanta, GA

3

COMPARISON OF BUSERELIN TO DANAZOL THERAPY IN ENDOMETRIOSIS

A. LEMAY and HRPI buserelin protocol 310 study group

Endocrinology of Reproduction, Hospital Saint-Francoise D'Assise, Quebec G1L 3L5, Canada;

Hoechst – Roussel Pharmaceuticals Inc. Somerville, New Jersey, USA and Hoechst Canada Inc. Montreal, Quebec, Canada

INTRODUCTION

Although the etiology of endometriosis is not understood, it is known that the ectopic endometrial tissue is sensitive to the production of sex steroid hormones during the menstrual cycle. Endometriosis is rare before menarche and develops usually during the reproductive years. The importance of ovarian steroids in the development and maintenance of endometriosis is also demonstrated by the usual curative effect of oophorectomy and the spontaneous regression of the disease at menopause. Experimentally implanted endometriosis in castrated monkeys requires sex steroids for its maintenance [1].

Although the glandular and epithelial cell morphology in the endometriotic tissue is heterogeneous, the majority of human endometriotic implants contain estrogen, progesterone and androgen receptors [2-5]. These findings can possibly explain the therapeutic effect of all three classes of steroid hormones as medical treatments for endometriosis. Since 1960, various high dosages of synthetic steroids have been used to treat endometriosis. In the 1960s and 1970s, the available hormonal treatments were continuous oral contraceptives (pseudopregnancy) and progestin-only regimens [6-7]. During the 1980s, danazol has become the primary hormonal agent in the treatment of endometriosis [8-10]. A hormonal milieu high in androgens or progestogens has a probable direct action on endometriotic implants but also induces a low estrogen environment by interfering with gonadotropin secretion and ovarian follicular development. Since steroid hormones have a multiplicity of effects, their mode of action is complex. They may also alter growth factors and immunological factors. Although they are generally well tolerated, steroid side effects are frequent and numerous.

In view of the hormone dependency of endometriosis, the possibility of selectively suppressing the ovarian secretion of estrogens by repetitive GnRH agonist administration is a new therapeutic approach for this disease. In the human, the main mechanism explaining the inhibitory effect of superactive GnRH agonists is a reversible down-regulation of gonadotropin secretion inducing a state of hypogonadotrophic hypogonadism (pseudomenopause or medical castration). In the recent literature, original papers have reported 6-month trials of several GnRH agonists in short series of patients with endometriosis proven at recent laparoscopy or laparotomy [11-19].

The purpose of this study was to evaluate the efficacy and safety of GnRH agonist treatment by comparison with conventional danazol therapy. A multicenter randomized standard control trial was initiated comparing buserelin with the usually recommended dosage regimen of danazol. The paper reports the preliminary analysis of data from 170 out of 330 patients who were enrolled into the study.

CLINICAL TRIAL PROTOCOL

Patients between the ages of 20 and 40 years were admitted to the study within 6 weeks after endometriosis was documented by laparoscopy or laparotomy and scored according to the revised American Fertility Society (AFS) classification [20]. Patients who had taken danazol within the last 6 months or oral contraceptives within the past 2 months, used a drug-releasing IUD within the past 3 months or had received any investigational drug within the last 4 weeks were excluded from enrolment into the study. Patients with other conditions in which danazol was contraindicated were also excluded. At the time of admission, patients signed an informed consent.

Patients were randomized to receive either buserelin treatment (n=118) or danazol treatment (n=52) in a ratio of 2 to 1. Once randomized to buserelin, the patient had the choice to receive the drug by intranasal insufflation (IN: 87 patients) or by subcutaneous injection (SC: 31 patients). The buserelin dosage for SC injection was 200µg once daily and, for intranasal administration, 400µg (2 sprays of 100µg in each nostril) given 3 times daily (every 8 hours).

Twenty-eight patients (53%) treated with danazol received the maximal dosage of 800mg/day (2 x 400mg/day or 4 x 200mg/day) at the start of treatment irrespective of the stage of endometriosis. A dosage of 400mg/day (2 x 200mg/day) of danazol was used in 11 patients presenting with mild to moderate endometriosis, accounting for 21.2% of the danazol treated patients. In the other 13 patients (25.0%) treated with danazol (mostly moderate cases), the dosage was increased from 400mg/day at the beginning of the treatment to 600mg/day and/or to 800mg/day during the treatment period. The decision to increase the danazol dosage was made by the treating physician based upon the clinical status of the patient.

The treatment was started between days 2 and 5 of menses and was administered for 6 months. In a limited number of cases where symptoms were improved but not cleared, the treatment was continued up to 9 months (12 buserelin cases and 6 danazol cases).

During the treatment period, patients were seen at the clinic at monthly intervals for clinical evaluation. Blood was then drawn for the determination of serum gonadotropins and estradiol levels. Hormones were measured by currently used radioimmunoassay techinques. Safety laboratory tests (hematology, urine analysis and serum biochemical tests) were evaluated every 2 months. At the end of the treatment, the endometriosis was reevaluated by laparoscopy and an optional endometrial biopsy was done. During a 6 month post-treatment follow-up, patients were seen at the clinic every 2 weeks for the first 2 months and every 2 months thereafter for repeated clinical, hormonal and biological evaluation.

One way analysis of variance was used to evaluate the changes from baseline values in the means of serum estradiol levels and serum cholesterol levels measured every treatment month within each group of patients. One way analysis of variance was also used to evaluate the differences in the means of the AFS scores between the buserelin and the danazol groups. The mean values of the 2 medications were analyzed at the beginning and at the end of treatment. Two way analysis of variance was used to compare the means of AFS scores within a single drug treatment. Pretreatment and posttreatment values were compared for total scores, implant scores and adhesion scores. The statistical significance of the changes in the means was calculated using the Duncan-Kramer multiple range test. The changes were considered significant when the P value was <0.05. The fluctuations in the number of patients available for a particular parameter are indicated in the text or in the tables.

The statistical analyses were done at St-Francois d'Assise Hospital on partial data sets which were not corrected for baseline variables e.g. race, age, stage of the disease, previous surgery on pelvic organs.

DECREASE IN SERUM ESTRADIOL LEVELS DURING TREATMENT

There was no statistical difference in the baseline values of serum estradiol between the different groups at the beginning of the treatment (Fig. 1). In the IN and SC buserelin groups, there was a progressive decrease in the mean circulating estradiol levels which were significantly lower than baseline at 1 month of treatment (P <0.01). Lower levels of serum estradiol were obtained with the SC route than with the IN route. However, a significant difference between the two buserelin curves was found only at 1 month (P <0.05).

At 400mg/day of danazol, there was no significant decrease in serum estradiol during the entire treatment period. When the dosage was increased from 400mg/day at the beginning of the treatment up to 800mg/day during the treatment, a significant decrease in the mean estradiol levels was observed at 6 months of treatment (P <0.05). At maximal dosage (800mg/day) from the start of the treatment, a significant decrease (P <0.05) in the mean serum estradiol levels was achieved at 3 and 4 months.

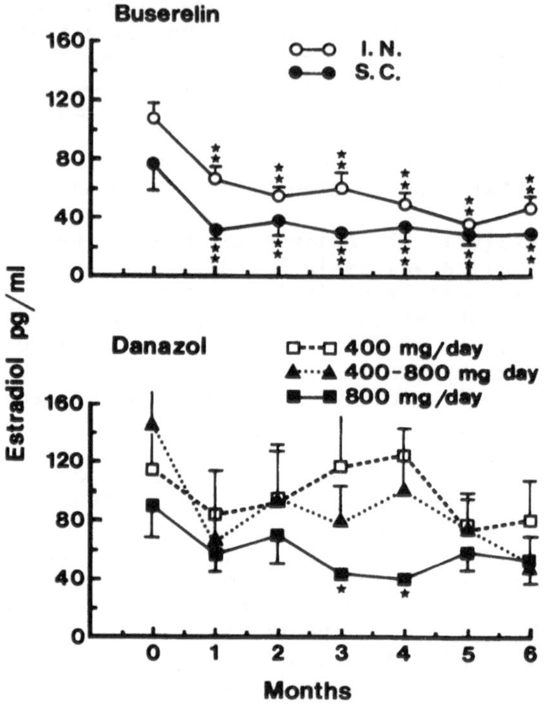

FIGURE 1. Means ± SEM of serum estradiol levels in the different medication groups on treatment day 1 and at monthly visits during hormonal therapy. *P <0.05 and **P <0.01 indicate levels of statistical significance for difference from pretreatment baseline within each estradiol curve.

The comparisons between the curves of the different dosage regimens indicate a better inhibition of serum estradiol by buserelin (IN or SC) compared to the high dose of danazol.

The inhibitory effect of danazol on ovarian steroidogenesis was smaller and less consistent when compared to that of buserelin. In this study, buserelin was effective in decreasing circulating FSH levels whereas no significant effect of danazol was found on serum FSH. No comments can be made about LH because the various centers have used different radioimmunoassay showing various correlations with the biological activity of LH. It is now well demonstrated that daily buserelin administration causes an important down-regulation of gonadotropin production [14, 17]. Previous studies have reported a weak or an inconsistent suppression of gonadotropins by danazol [21-23]. Thus, the absence of marked decreases in circulating estradiol in the danazol groups would be related to the poor inhibitory effect of the drug on gonadotropin secretion.

IMPROVEMENT IN SYMPTOMS AND SIGNS

The results have been combined for all the symptomatic cases in the buserelin groups as compared to the total number of danazol patients presenting endometriosis symptoms. A higher percentage of women reported a disappearance or an alleviation of dyspareunia and intermenstrual pelvic pain during danazol treatment than during buserelin treatment. However, at physical examination

Table 1. Effect of buserelin and danazol on the incidence of endometriosis symptoms at the end of the treatment.

Symptoms	BUSERELIN		DANAZOL	
	Before Treatment Patients n (%)	End of Treatment Patients n (%)	Before Treatment Patients n (%)	End of Treatment Patients n (%)
DYSPAREUNIA				
none	36 (49.3)	58 (79.4)	20 (55.5)	32 (88.9)
mild	21 (28.7)	10 (13.7)	9 (25.0)	2 (5.6)
moderate	12 (16.4)	3 (4.1)	5 (13.9)	0 (0.0)
severe	4 (5.5)	2 (2.7)	2 (5.5)	1 (2.8)
PELVIC PAIN				
none	33 (43.4)	58 (76.3)	14 (37.8)	34 (91.9)
mild	25 (32.9)	16 (21.0)	15 (40.5)	3 (8.1)
moderate	18 (23.7)	1 (1.3)	8 (21.6)	0 (0.0)
PELVIC TENDERNESS				
none	32 (42.1)	66 (86.8)	12 (33.3)	28 (77.8)
mild	31 (40.8)	9 (11.8)	19 (52.8)	8 (22.2)
moderate	13 (17.1)	0 (0.0)	5 (13.9)	0 (0.0)
PELVIC INDURATION				
none	44 (57.9)	64 (84.2)	22 (61.1)	23 (63.9)
mild	21 (27.6)	11 (14.5)	7 (19.4)	10 (27.8)
moderate	9 (11.8)	1 (1.3)	6 (16.7)	3 (8.3)
severe	2 (2.6)	0 (0.0)	1 (2.8)	0 (0.0)

pelvic tenderness and pelvic induration were improved more with buserelin than with danazol. Little or no pain was associated with the breakthrough bleeding which occurred during the treatment period. Consequently, both drugs have good efficacy in alleviating the clinical symptoms and signs of endometriosis during treatment.

IMPROVEMENT IN AFS SCORES AT LAPAROSCOPY

Before treatment, the total AFS point score was not significantly higher in the buserelin group compared to the danazol group. There

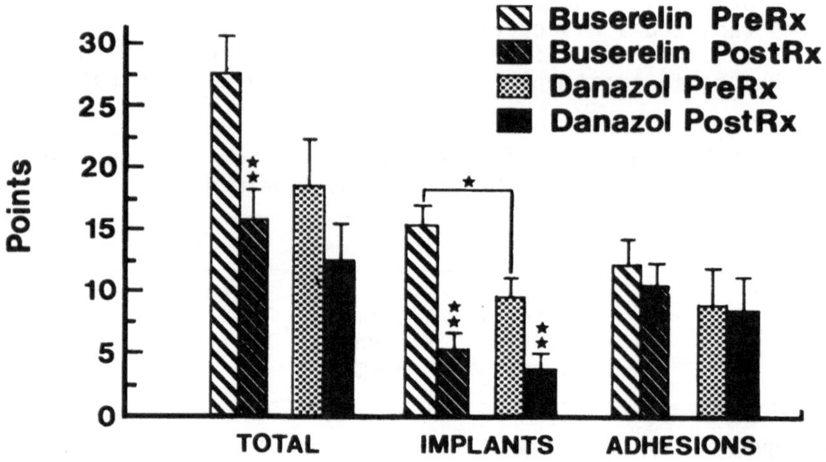

FIGURE 2 Means ± SEM of points of ASF endometriosis scores for the combined groups of buserelin and danazol treatment patients at all stages before treatment and at the end of treatment. *P <0.05 indicates the statistical difference between the implant scores of the buserelin and danazol groups before treatment **P <0.01 indicates level of statistical significance for posttretment values compared to pretreatment values within each drug treatment group.

was no difference in the adhesion scores between the 2 groups but the mean implant score at first laparoscopy was significantly higher (P <0.05) in the buserelin group than in the danazol group.

At the end of the treatment, there was a significant decrease (P <0.01) in the mean total score of the buserelin group. No significant diminution was found in the danazol group. There was no effect of either treatment on the means of adhesion scores. Thus, the overall improvement in total score was attributed to the effect of treatment on the implant scores. Both medications were effective in causing a significant reduction (P <0.01) in the mean implant score compared to pretreatment. The initial implant score was significantly higher (P <0.05) in the buserelin group than in the danazol group. However, the reduction in implant score was greater with buserelin than with danazol.

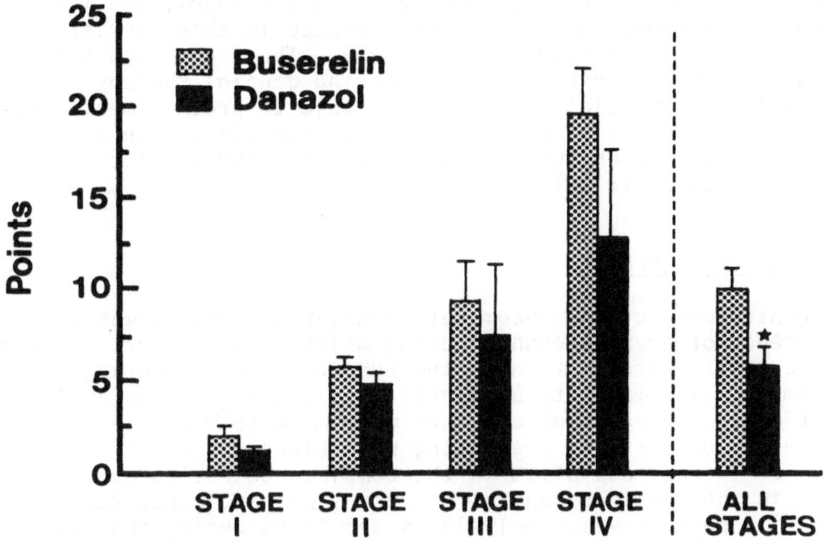

FIGURE 3 Means ± SEM of points of endometriosis implants that were reduced from baseline at the end of buserelin and danazol treatment for each stage and all the stages combined. *P <0.05 indicates the level of significance of difference between buserelin and danazol for all stages combined.

Buserelin also caused a greater reduction than danazol in mean implant points at each stage (Fig. 3). When the reduction was calculated as a percentage of baseline, the reduction was always greater in the buserelin groups than in the danazol groups for each stage. In stages I and II, 50% of the patients did not have the maximal danazol dosage which could account for the lesser efficacy of danazol. However, in stages III and IV the highest danazol dosage was compared to buserelin and there was also a greater reduction in implant scores with buserelin compared to danazol. When all the stages were combined, the difference in implant reduction was significant ($P < 0.05$).

Although the drug used was known to the laparoscopist and these preliminary results have not been corrected for differences in baseline variables, the data of this multicenter trial indicate a better efficacy for buserelin than danazol in reducing the active part of the disease. Since endometriosis tissue is mainly estrogen dependent, this better efficacy could be explained by the better ability of the buserelin treatment to decrease serum estradiol. Although serum estradiol was also decreased with the higher dosage regimen for danazol, the inhibition was not as good as, or as consistent as, that observed with buserelin. It has been demonstrated that during danazol treatment, the levels of sex hormone binding globulin (SHBG) carrying estradiol, are markedly decreased as compared to a slight increase in this carrier protein in a GnRH agonist treated patient [25]. Thus, although serum estradiol appears to be decreased during danazol therapy, free or bioavailable estradiol remains comparable to pretreatment levels with this medication. Mechanisms of action other than estrogen inhibition have been invoked to explain the therapeutic effect of danazol on endometriosis.

CLINICAL SIDE EFFECTS

One consequence of the incomplete ovarian inhibition was the occurrence of breakthrough bleeding which occurred more frequently in the danazol groups than in the buserelin groups during treatment. The majority of bleeding episodes happened during the first month of treatment and they were mild to moderate. The percentage of patients presenting with bleeding during the first month of therapy was 57.5% in the combined buserelin groups and 62.0% in the combined danazol groups. This incidence decreased with time being respectively 13.7% and 20.9% during the last month of treatment. The overall incidences of bleeding calculated on a monthly basis for the 6 months of treatment were 28.2% and 27.4%

Table 2. Percentage of patients presenting most significant side effects possibly or probably related to study drug.

Side effect	BUSERELIN	DANAZOL
	Patients n (%)	Patients n (%)
Hot flushes	82 (70.7)	18 (35.3)
Vaginal dryness	34 (29.3)	4 (7.8)
Decreased libido	11 (9.5)	5 (9.8)
Weight gain	1 (0.9)	22 (43.1)
Oedema	2 (1.7)	17 (33.3)
Myalgia	2 (1.7)	12 (23.5)
Arthralgia	3 (2.6)	2 (3.9)
Increased appetite	0 (0.0)	3 (5.9)
Nausea	4 (3.4)	6 (11.8)
Acne	7 (6.0)	16 (31.4)
Hirsutism	2 (1.7)	5 (9.8)
Alopecia	0 (0.0)	5 (9.8)
Breast atrophy	2 (1.7)	6 (11.8)
Asthenia	8 (6.9)	17 (33.3)
Headache	27 (23.3)	8 (15.7)
Migraine	5 (4.3)	2 (3.9)
Emotional lability	7 (6.0)	11 (21.6)
Depression	5 (4.3)	2 (3.9)

in the groups treated with buserelin (IN and SC), the respective frequencies of uterine bleeding per month for low, intermediate, and high dosages of danazol were 51.6%, 49.4% and 22.1%. The incidence of severe bleeding varied between 0.9% to 2% in all the dosage groups except for danazol 800mg where it was 6.6%. Bleeding was considered severe not because of excessive amount but because it occurred daily for prolonged periods or throughout the month.

Clinical side effects of both medications have been reported in previous studies [9, 10, 14, 15, 18]. Table 2 lists the most significant clinical side effects to be compared in the present study and that were possibly or probably related to the study drug. In the buserelin group, hot flushes were frequent and often moderate to severe whereas in the danazol group, they were less frequent and mainly mild to moderate. In the buserelin group, sexually active women reported lack of adequate vaginal secretion at the time of intercourse. The libido was frequently decreased in these women. The decreased libido in the danazol group was apparently not related to decreased vaginal secretion.

The side effects caused by danazol were mainly related to the anabolic action (weight gain, oedema, myalgia, increased appetite) and androgenic action (acne, hirsutism, alopecia) of the steroid derivative. It is interesting to note that the incidence of breast atrophy was only 1.7% in the buserelin group as compared to 11.8% in the danazol group. This finding would indicate that the regression of breast tissue would not be related to the estrogen deprivation alone but would rather be related to an androgenic milieu.

It is also interesting to consider that nausea, asthenia and emotional lability were 3 to 5 times more frequent during danazol therapy than during buserelin therapy. On the other hand, there was a significant occurrence of headaches which were more frequent in the buserelin groups (23.3%) than in the danazol group (15.7%). The percentage of migraine was low and comparable in both groups. The percentage of depression was also comparable in both groups for buserelin and danazol respectively (4.3 and 3.9%). Depression can be a serious side effect. The history of previous depression should be considered before treatment in order to avoid any potential major complications.

In this research study, the menopausal symptoms induced by buserelin were frequent but in general were well accepted. However, the anabolic effects and the androgenic signs caused by danazol were also frequent and often of great concern to the patients.

LABORATORY SAFETY TESTS

Laboratory tests including hemogram, urinalysis and usual serum biochemical tests were evaluated every 2 months during the treatment period and at 2 and 6 months in the post-treatment period. These data have not been analyzed yet but remained in the normal range in the individual patients. In previous reports on buserelin treatment, there were no significant changes in usual

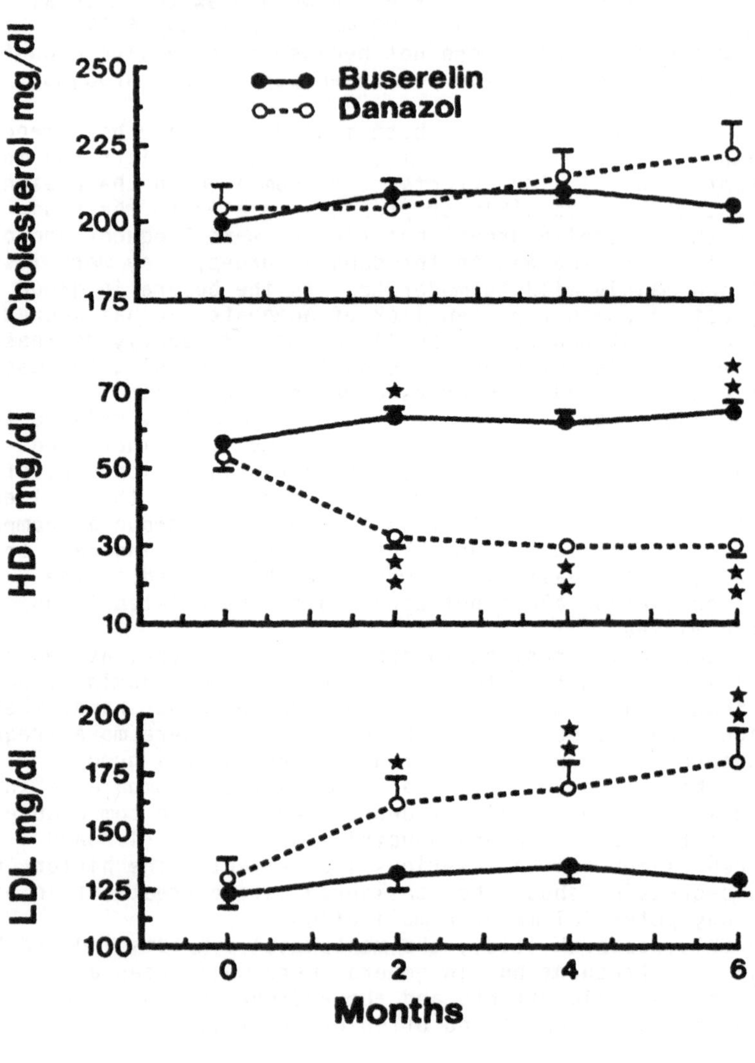

FIGURE 4 Means ± SEM of serum cholesterol, HDL- cholesterol and LDL- cholesterol values for the combined groups of buserelin and of danazol patients. *P <0.05 and ** P <0.01 indicate levels of statistical significance for difference from pretreatment baseline within each dosage curve.

laboratory tests when evaluated at similar time intervals [14, 18]. High dose danazol treatment was shown to be associated with mild elevations of SGPT, SGOT, LDH and CPK which resolve spontaneously after cessation of treatment [26].

In this report, we compared the effects of buserelin and danazol on serum cholesterol and its high density lipoprotein (HDL) and low density lipoprotein (LDL) subfractions. There were no apparent differences in mean cholesterol values between the various dosage groups for either buserelin or danazol.

For total cholesterol, values were available for 105 buserelin and 49 danazol patients at admission. At the end of the treatment, the number of patients were 91 and 42 respectively. For lipoprotein subfractions, the numbers of patients evaluated were 67 and 31 for buserelin and danazol at admission. These figures were respectively 57 and 26 at the end of the treatment.

The total cholesterol in the danazol group increased but not significantly during treatment (Fig. 4). However, danazol treatment caused a marked and significant decrease in HDL-cholesterol ($P < 0.01$) after 2 months of treatment. These low levels of HDL-cholesterol masked a significant increase in LDL-cholesterol ($P < 0.05$ at month 2, $P < 0.01$ at months 4 and 6). In the buserelin treated patients, there was a non significant increase in LDL and total cholesterol. However, the increase in LDL-cholesterol was compensated by a small but significant increase in HDL-cholesterol, ($P < 0.05$). Total cholesterol and its subfractions returned to pretreatment levels at 2 months after discontinuation of treatment. These changes in cholesterol metabolism would be of concern for patients with elevated cholesterol levels and for chronic treatment since the risk of coronary heart disease is proportional to the level of LDL-cholesterol and inversely related to HDL-cholesterol levels. These preliminary results appear to indicate a safety advantage for buserelin over danazol.

One potential disadvantage of estrogen deprivation would be accelerated bone loss. Recent reports on GnRH agonist treatment of endometriosis indicated an increase in urinary calcium-creatinine ratio [18]. A small decrease of the trabecular bone of the lumbar vertebrae was estimated by computed tomography after 6 months of treatment [27, 28]. There was a small decrease in the bone mineral content in the trabecular zone of the lumbar vertebrae measured by dual photon absorptiometry [29]. However, there were no significant changes in the cortical zone of the mid-shaft of the femur and of the radius evaluated respectively by dual and single photon absorptiometry [28, 29]. The reported changes appear to be readily reversible after discontinuation of treatment. The bone loss is small and reversible; thus the administration of this GnRH agonist for a period of 6 months should not adversely affect eumonorrheic woman with a normal bone mass.

RETURN OF MENSES AND FERTILITY

The mean time interval between cessation of treatment and first uterine bleeding varied with the different drug regimens. It was 47.6±2.3 days and 50.0 + 3.5 days in the 2 buserelin groups (IN: n=72; SC: n=20). The time-intervals in the danazol groups were shorter, being 31.9±1.8 days for the 400mg/day dose (n=8), 37.9±5.9 days for the 400 to 800mg/day dose (n=12) and 40.1±3.0 days for the 800mg/day dose (n=17). These results indicate that the time required to reactivate the pituitary-ovarian function was proportional to the degree of estrogen suppression by buserelin and danazol. The amount and duration of menses were reported as normal.

At the time of the second laparoscopy, no major surgery was done although occasionally an implant was biopsied or an adhesion broken during organ manipulation. In a limited number of cases, a laser was used to vaporize implants or free adhesions. These isolated complementary actions would not have a significant effect on the overall preliminary evaluation of the follow-up.

The dysmenorrhea associated with endometriosis before treatment disappeared or was diminished in severity at the time of the return of the menses. The number of patients presenting with this symptom before treatment was 92 in the buserelin group and 39 in the danazol group for a respective incidence of 90.0% and 94.7%. At 6 months post-treatment, the respective numbers of cases evaluated (excluding pregnancies) were 61 and 27. At the end of 6 months of follow-up, the percentage of patients free of dysmenorrhea was 29.5% in the buserelin groups and 25.9% in the danazol groups. The percentage of moderate and severe dysmenorrhea decreased from 27.2% and 30.4% to 6.6% and 16.4% in the buserelin groups. In the danazol groups, the corresponding incidence decreased from 18.4% and 31.6% to 11.1% and 7.4%. For mild dysmenorrhea, the incidence increased from 31.0% to 47.5% in the buserelin treated patients and from 44.7% to 55.6% in the danazol treated patients. The increased incidence of mild dysmenorrhea is obviously related to the incomplete improvement in patients complaining of moderate and severe dysmenorrhea before treatment. During the first 6 months of follow-up, the other endometriosis symptoms were also decreased in a comparable manner.

Numerous pregnancies have occurred within 6 months following the discontinuation of therapy. The proportion of pregnancies appear to be equivalent between the 2 treatment groups. In the number of pregnancies evauated, the incidence of abortion was low and the completion of pregnancies with normal children was high. A much greater number of patients over a longer period of time will be required to properly assess the numerous factors implicated in fertility.

CONCLUDING REMARKS

Although the results of this multicenter control led trial are incomplete and preliminary, it is clear that buserelin could be an advantageous alternative to danazol for the medical treatment of endometriosis. Buserelin has a better efficacy in inhibiting ovarian steroidogenesis and in inducing a consistent but relative hypoestrogenic state. At posttreatment laparoscopic evaluation, a greater reduction in the mean score of the active implants has been found with buserelin than with danazol. The relief of symptoms appeared similar with both drugs. Although the incidence of side effects was similar between the 2 groups, those reported for the danazol patients tended to be more serious and less acceptable to the patients. The patients were less concerned with the menopausal sysmptoms associated with buserelin than with the anabolic and androgenic effects caused by danazol. According to serum biochemical tests, buserelin could be a safer drug than danazol. The elevation of LDL-cholesterol caused by danazol should be considered as a cautionary note for patients having hypercholesterolemia or requiring repeated or chronic treatment (>6 months). Although with buserelin the bone loss has been reported to be small and reversible, further studies are required to evaluate this aspect especially for prolonged dosing in patients requiring repeated or chronic treatment. The recent development of monthly depot delivery systems such as biodegradable implants injected SC and biodegradable microcapsules injected IM should increase the practicability, the compliance and the efficacy of this new class of medication.

ACKNOWLEDGEMENTS

To Sol S. Klioze, Ph.D, for data collection and revision to Lucile T. Lemay, M.D., Ph.D, for data tabulation, graphics and statistical analysis and to Louise Mercier for typing the manuscript.

The HRPI buserelin protocol 310 study group members were:

M. Yusoff Dawood, MD, Department of Obstetrics and Gynecology, University of Illinois at Chicago, College of Medicine, Chicago, Illinois. W. Paul Dmowski, MD, Rush-Presbyterian St. Lukes Medical Center, Chicago, Illinois; R. Donald Gambrell, Jr. MD, Robert B. Greenblatt, MD, Greenblatt and Gambrell Clinic, Augusta, Georgia; Andre Lemay, MD, PhD, Department d'obstetrique- gynecologie, Hopital Saint-Francois d'Assise, Universite Laval, Quebec, Quebec, Canada; Daniel R. Mishell, MD, Women's Hospital, Los Angeles, California; Manubai Nagamani, MD, Department of Obstetrics and Gynecology, University of Texas Medical Branch, Galveston, Texas; Roger J. Pepperell, MD, The Royal Woman's Hospital, Carlton, Victoria, Australia; Robert W. Shaw, MD, Head of Obstetrics and Gynecology, The Royal Free Hospital, London, England; Machelle M. Seibel, MD, Boston Center for Reproductive

Health, Boston, Massachusetts; Steven J. Sondheimer, MD, Department of Obstetrics and Gynecology, Hospital of the University of Pennsylvania, Philadelphia, Pennsylvania; Sol S. Klioze, PhD, Charles Matthijssen, PhD, Timothy P. Spiro, MD, Hoechst-Roussel Pharmaceuticals Inc., Somerville, New Jersey; Patrick Merat, MD, Hoechst Canada Inc., Montreal, Quebec, Canada.

REFERENCES

1. Dizerega, GS, Barber, DL, and Hodgen, GD (1980). Endometriosis: Role of ovarian steroids in initiation, maintenance and suppression. Fertil Steril, 33, 649
2. Bergquist, A, Ljungberg, O, and Myhre, E (1984). Comparison of the histological appearance of human endometrium and endometriotic tissue obtained simultaneously: A preliminary report. Acta Obstet Gynecol Scand (Suppl), 123, 11
3. Janne, O, Kauppila, A, and Kokko, E (1981). Estrogen and progestin receptors in endometriotic lesions: comparison with endometrial tissue. Am J Obstet Gynecol, 141, 562
4. Tamaya, T, Motoyama, T, and Ohono, Y (1979). Steroid receptor levels and histology of endometriosis and adenomysis. Fertil Steril, 31, 396
5. Vihko, R, Isotalo, H, and Kauppila, A (1984). Hormonal regulation of endometrium and endometriosis tissue. In: Raynaud, JP (ed.) "Medical Management of Endometriosis". p 79. (New York: Raven Press)
6. Kistner, RW (1958). The use of newer progestins in the treatment of endometriosis. Am J Obstet Gynecol, 75, 264
7. Kistner, RW (1959). The treatment of endometriosis by inducing pseudopregnancy with ovarian hormones: a report of 58 cases. Fertil Steril, 10, 539
8. Dmowski, WP, and Cohen, MR (1978). Antigonadotropin (danazol) in the treatment of endometriosis. Am J Obstet Gynecol, 130, 41
9. Barbieri, RL, Evans, S, and Kistner, RW (1982). Danazol in the treatment of endometriosis: analysis of of 100 cases with a 4-year follow-up. Fertil Steril, 36, 737
10. Buttram, VC, Reiter, RC, and Ward, S (1985). Treatment of endometriosis with danazol: report of a six year prospective study. Fertil Steril, 43, 353
11. Lemay, A, and Quesnel, G (1982). Potential new treament of endometriosis: reversible inhibition of pituitary-ovarian function by chronic intranasal administration of a luteinizing hormone-releasing hormone (LH-RH) agonist. Fertil Steril, 38, 376
12. Shaw, RW, Fraser, HM, and Boyle, H (1983). Intranasal treatment with luteinizing hormone releasing hormone agonist in women with endometriosis. Brit Med J, 287, 1667
13. Pring, DW, Maresh, M, and Fraser, AC (1983). Luteinizing hormone releasing hormone agonist in women with endometriosis. Brit Med J, 287, 1718

14. Lemay, A, Maheux, R, Faure, N, Jean, C, and Fazekas, ATA (1984). Reversible hypogonadism induced by a luteinizing hormone-releasing hormone (LH-RH) agonist (buserelin) as a new therapeutic approach for endometriosis. Fertil Steril, 41, 863
15. Schriock, E, Monroe, SE, Henzl, M, and Jaffe, RB (1985). Treatment of endometriosis with a potent agonist of gonadotropin-releasing hormone (nafarelin). Fertil Steril, 44, 583
16. Zorn, JR, Tanger, Ch, Roger, M, Grenier, J, Comaru-Schally, AM, and Schally, AV (1986). Therapeutic hypogonadism induced by a delayed-release preparation of microcapsules of D-Trp-6-luteinizing hormone-releasing hormone: A preliminary study in eight women with endometriosis. Int J Fertil, 3, 11
17. Hardt, W, Schimdt-Gollwitzer, M, Schmidt-Gollwitzer K, Genz, T, and Nevinny-Stickel, J (1986). Erst ergebnisse bei der behandlung der endometriose mit dem LH-RH-analogon buserelin. Geburtsh u Frauenheilk, 46, 483
18. Steingold, KA, Cedars, M, Ju, JKH, Randle, D, Judd, HL, and Meldrum, DR (1987). Treatment of endometriosis with a long-acting gonadotropin-releasing hormone agonist. Obstet Gynecol, 69, 403
19. Lemay, A, Maheux, R, Huot, C, Blanchet, J, and Faure, N (1988). Efficacy of intranasal or subcutaneous luteinizing hormone- releasing hormone agonist inhibition of ovarian function in the treatment of endometriosis. Am J Obstet Gynecol (in press)
20. American Fertility Society (1979). Classification of endometriosis. Fertil Steril, 32, 633
21. Fraser, IS, Markham, R, McIlveen, J, and Robinson, M (1982). Dynamic tests of hypothalamic and pituitary function in women treated with danazol. Fertil Steril 37, 484
22. Dmowski, PW, Headley, S, and Radwanska, E (1983). Effects of danazol on pulsatile gonadotropin patterns and on serum estradiol levels in normally cycling women. Fertil Steril, 39, 49
23. Rannevik, G, and Thorell, JI (1984). The influence of danazol on pituitary function and on the ovarian follicular hormone secretion in premenopausal women. Acta Obstet Gynecol Scand (Suppl), 123, 89
24. Hardt, W, and Schmidt-Gollwitzer, M (1983). Sustained gonadal suppression in fertile women with the LHRH agonist buserelin. Clin Endocrinol, 19, 613
25. Meldrum, DR, Pardridge, WM, Karow, WG, Rivier, J, Vale, W, and Judd, HL (1983). Hormonal effects of danazol and medical oophorectomy in endometriosis. Obstet Gynecol, 62, 480
26. Holt, JP, and Keller, D (1984). Danazol treatment increases serum enzyme levels. Fertil Steril, 41, 70
27. Cann, CE, Henzl, M, Burry, K, Andreko, J, Hanson, F, Adamson, D, Trobough, G, and Strewler, G (1986). Reversible bone loss is induced by GnRH agonist. 68th Annual Meeting of the Endocrine Society, Anaheim, California, Abstract
28. Matta, WH, Shaw, RW, Hesp, R, and Katz, D (1987). Hypogonadism induced by luteinizing hormone releasing hormone agonist analogues: effects on bone density in premenopausal women. Brit Med J, 294, 1523
29. Devogelaer, JP, DeDeuxchaisnes, CN, Donnez, J, and Thomas, K (1987). LHRH analogues and bone loss. The Lancet, I, 1498

4

LHRH AGONIST TREATMENT OF ENDOMETRIOSIS

Angelo CONTI
Ch. de Mornex 6, 1003 Lausanne, Switzerland

INTRODUCTION

Endometriosis is a common disease in women during the reproductive ages. Estimates of the frequency of endometriosis range from 3% to 20% of the white female population and it is certainly the most prominent gynecological entity after uterine fibroids. Present therapeutic modalities for endometriosis include conservative surgery or ovarian suppression with hormones. The use of medical treatments is directed towards achieving ovarian suppression to avoid the steroidal stimulation of ectopic endometrial tissues.

The objectives of this study were to evaluate the clinical effectiveness, safety and tolerance of 6 months of treatment with intranasal buserelin. Patients were selected for laparoscopy from those with sterility problems or with other symptoms suggesting endometriosis. Laparoscopy and dye hydrotubation were performed on subfertile patients without other signs or symptoms suggestive of endometriosis. Women who satisfied the following criteria were admitted to the trial: 1. Age between 18 and 40 years; 2. Having a spontaneous menstrual cycle; 3. Endometriosis confirmed by laparoscopy. The following patients were excluded: 1. Those who had received danazol or hormonal treatment without success: 2. If they had received danazol within the previous 6 months; 3. If they received drugs which might interfere with evaluation of the response to the therapy; 4. If they had mild endometriosis.

PATIENTS AND PROTOCOL

Of the 12 patients reported in this study, 8 received buserelin because of involuntary infertility and 4 because of dysmenorrhea, dyspareunia or because of intermenstrual pelvic pain. When scored according to the American Fertility Society (AFS) classification for implants and adhesions, 7 women were classified as having moderate, 4 as having severe and 1 as having extensive endometriosis. Eleven women completed 6 months treatment and reported satisfactory compliance.

A total dose of 900 µg per day was administered by insufflation of 1 spray in each nostril at 8 hour intervals. This buserelin dose was chosen although we were fully aware of the fact that it produces only a partial suppression of the ovarian function related to the degree of inhibition of serum gonadotropins. Although previous results had clearly shown that starting treatment in the luteal phase avoids the initial estrogen elevation, we decided to start buserelin treatment in all patients within the first 3 days of the follicular phase. This was due to the fact that a majority of the patients entering this study were infertility patients; a beginning pregnancy had to be ruled out with absolute criteria. Any changes in symptoms, physical signs, bleeding pattern or side effects were recorded. Physical examination and complete hematology and serum biochemistry were performed before starting the treatment and at the end. At monthly intervals blood samplings were obtained for evaluation of LH, FSH, estradiol (E2) and progesterone (P) by radioimmunoassays. A second laparoscopy was performed on the last day of therapy.

RESULTS

The hormonal response to buserelin treatment is shown in Figure 1. With prolonged treatment, the mean LH concentration showed a slight decrease compared with a baseline level of 12.3 ± 3.8 IU/l measured on 1 of the first 3 days of the menstrual

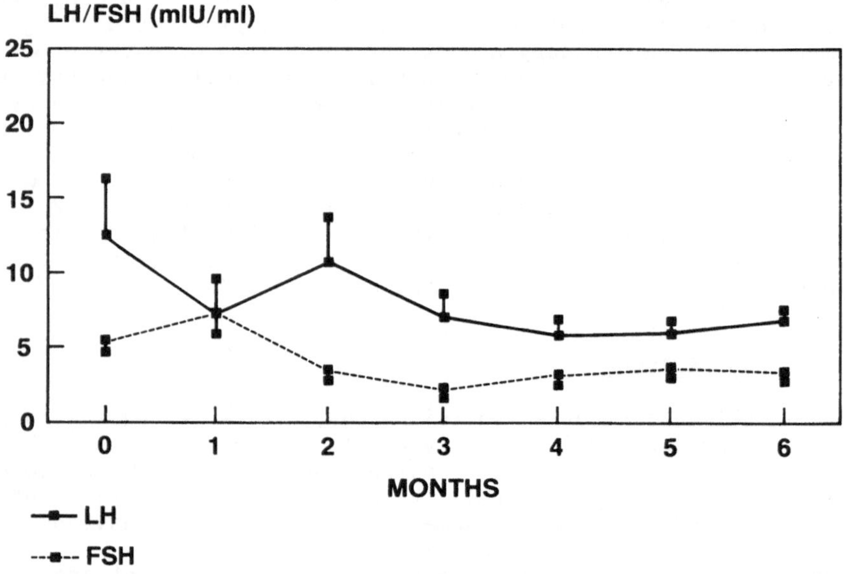

FIGURE 1 LH and FSH levels (mean±SEM) 12 patients treated withbuserelin

period. The mean starting FSH level of 5.4 ± 0.7 IU/l remained unaltered after the first month but decreased thereafter to values around 3.5 IU/l. Figure 2 shows the ovarian suppression due to gonadotropin inhibition. Before starting buserelin, E2 was 444 ± 122 pmol/l; after 1 month of therapy, the E2 values recorded were widely scattered. Four patients still had pre-treatment levels; 4 patients had only a slight decrease of E2 and only 4 out of 12 patients had an E2 definitely below early follicular phase

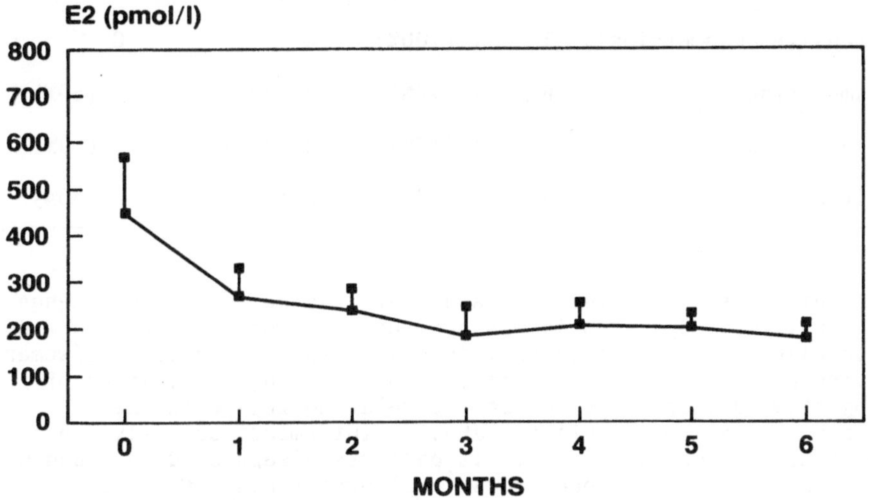

FIGURE 2 E2 levels (mean±SEM) in 12 patients treated with buserelin

range. The mean E2 of all 12 patients after 1 month was 267 ± 61 pmol/l, a value in the low range for the early follicular phase. From the third month onwards mean E2 remained just above the menopausal range. Progesterone concentrations remained low during the whole treatment period, indicating anovulation.

EFFICACY ON ENDOMETRIOSIS

The upper part of Table 1 shows the findings of the second laparoscopy. Two out of 12 patients were healed completely and both belonged to the group with moderate endometriosis. In all 4 patients having severe endometriosis, there was a reduction in the diameter of implants and in 3 the disappearance of some smaller foci. The only patient in this study having extensive endometriosis and very severe adhesions showed no improvement of AFS score at laparoscopy. The effects of 900 μg/day of buserelin on signs and symptoms have been tabulated in the lower part of Table 1. Before treatment 8 patients complained of severe dysmenorrhea; after 6 months this symptom had disappeared in 4

Table 1. Effect of buserelin treatment on signs and symptoms on endometriosis.

Sign/Symptom	n	No Change	Alleviated	Disappeared
Moderate endometriosis	7	0	5 (71%)	2 (29%)
Severe endometriosis	4	1 (25%)	3 (75%)	0
Extensive endometriosis	1	1 (100%)	0	0
Dysmenorrhea	8	1 (12%)	3 (38%)	4 (50%)
Dyspareunia	6	1 (17%)	2 (33%)	3 (50%)
Pelvic pain	5	1 (20%)	2 (40%)	2 (40%)

patients, was alleviated in 3 and there was no subjective change in 1 patient. Dyspareunia was present in 6 women before starting buserelin; it disappeared only in 50% of the patients. The woman having extensive endometriosis did not have any alleviation of subjective disturbances, a fact correlating well with the unchanged AFS score mentioned above. Intermenstrual pelvic pain which was present in 5 out of 12 patients disappeared in 2 and was alleviated in 2. Although occasional breast discomfort was reported at 2 or 3 weeks of treatment (probably related to the transient E2 elevation), buserelin had a beneficial effect on several patients who had breast tenderness before treatment.

An endometrial curettage was performed at the time of the second laparoscopy in all 12 patients. Blood only or debris were found in 60% of the curettings. Atrophic changes similar to those seen in the early menopause were observed in 33% of the specimens. Thin endometrial glands were scattered in a dense cellular stroma in these patients. In the last 2 biopsies, the endometrium was described as proliferative. There was no definite correlation between these results and the E2 levels measured the same day in individual patients.

SIDE EFFECTS AND SAFETY

Possible side effects had been discussed with all patients in a detailed way just before asking their formal consent. From the side effects reported in Table 2, only the hot flushes, which occurred in all patients, were subjectively a significant problem. The frequency of these hot flushes ranged from 2 per month to more than 15 per day. Vaginal dryness was noticed by 50% of these women. Although all patients had been encouraged to restrict their caloric intake from the beginning, 5 of 12 had a weight increase between 1 and 3 kilos. Beside the hot flushes the

Table 2. Side effects under buserelin treatment (n=12).

Side Effect	Incidence
Hot flushes	12 (100%)
Vaginal dryness	6 (50%)
Psychic alterations	5 (41%)
Weight gain	5 (41%)
Headaches	4 (33%)
Tiredness	3 (25%)
Breast discomfort during 1st month	3 (25%)
Changing of the skin	2 (16%)
Insomnia	1 (8%)

headaches seemed to be the most disturbing sign; the headaches became so intolerable for 1 patient that she decided to stop treatment after 4 months. Table 3 shows the bleeding pattern during buserelin treatment. Three out of 12 patients did not menstruate after starting treatment. Fifty percent of the women had bleeding within or at the end of the first month but no bleeding thereafter with the daily dose of 900 µg. Spotting was recorded by 5 patients and 2 of them also belonged to the group with bleedings within the first month. We had advised all our patients to increase the buserelin dose by 300 µg/day if bleeding episodes occurred after the first month. Three of them had to increase their daily regimen to stop bleedings; one went up

Table 3. Vaginal bleeding during buserelin treatment (n=12).

Bleeding Pattern	Incidence
Amenorrhea from first month	3 (25%)
Bleeding within first month	6 (50%)
Spotting	5 (41%)
Frequent bleedings with increase of the dose up to 1800 µ/day	3 (25%)

to a dose of 1200 µg, one to 1500 and the third one to 1800 µg/day. Side effects reported by these 3 patients were in the same range as the 9 other patients using the lower daily regimen.

Laboratory tests including hemograms and complete serum biochemistry were within the normal range in all 12 patients at the end of the treatment.

CONCLUSIONS

Three times daily intranasal insufflation of buserelin was effective in lowering serum estradiol to below the early follicular phase range. Our 3 patients with daily doses higher than 900 µg had a greater degree of ovarian suppression, but their side effects were in the same range than those reported by the other 9 patients. Although the numbers are small there seemed a correlation between the degree of E2 suppression and the disappearance of endometrial foci at laparoscopy.

Of the 4 patients having a delayed ovarian suppression three were definitely over-weight by more than 20%; a standard regimen of 900 µg/day does not have the capacity to produce the desired degree of ovarian suppression for obtaining satisfactory results.

We think that 1200 µg/day of buserelin should be the standard dose for all patients and that the treatment period needs to be prolonged to 9 or even 12 months in some patients with moderate or severe endometriosis.

This new endometriosis treatment appears to be very promising because of its lack of major subjective side effects, and because of its specificity and its rapid reversibility.

5

A PHASE III CLINICAL TRIAL OF BUSERELIN VERSUS DANAZOL IN THE TREATMENT OF ENDOMETRIOSIS

Wassim H.M. MATTA and **Robert W. SHAW**
The Academic Department of Obstetrics and Gynaecology
at The Royal Free Hospital School of Medicine,
London, NW3 2QG, UK

INTRUDUCTION

Hormonal treatments for endometriosis which are aimed at suppressing the pituitary-ovarian function ('pseudomenopause') seem to be superior to those regimes aimed at inducing a 'pseudopregnancy' state. Hypo-oestrogenism can cause atrophy and regression of endometriotic tissue.

Danazol therapy has been widely used in the treatment of endometriosis. One of its several presumed modes of action is the ability to reduce ovarian oestrogen secretion. This form of therapy is associated with a high incidence of troublesome side-effects [1].

The chronic administration of gonadotrophin releasing hormone (GnRH) agonists induces a reversible state of hypogonadotrophic hypogonadism, with resultant hypo-oestrogenism. Early reports [2, 3] on the use of the GnRH agonist, buserelin ($[D\text{-}Ser(TBU)^{6}]$LHRH ethylamide, Hoechst Pharmaceuticals), have been encouraging.

We present our preliminary results of a randomised, open-label, prospective clinical trial comparing buserelin, administered intranasally, to danazol, administered orally, in terms of their endocrine effects, clinical efficacy, patient tolerance and safety.

PATIENTS AND METHODS

Sixty patients aged 21 to 40 years were recruited into the study. Endometriosis was diagnosed and scored, according to the revised American Fertility Society (A.F.S.) classification [4], by laparoscopy within six weeks prior to onset of therapy. Patients were excluded from participation in the study if they had received danazol within six months or other sex steroid hormones within three months prior to entry. Following laparoscopy patients were randomised, by open-label, to receive either buserelin (n=40) or danazol (n=20). Treatment commenced on day 1 to 4 of the menstrual cycle, and continued for six months, at the end of which a second laparoscopic assessment and scoring was carried out. Subjects were followed up for a further six months after discontinuation of treatment. Each patient allocated to buserelin therapy received a fixed dose of 400μg t.i.d., intranasally. Patients randomised to danazol received 400-800mg total daily oral dose, depending on the severity of endometriosis and patient's response, in accordance with the package insert. Throughout treatment and follow up periods, patients were reviewed for clinical, endocrine and various safety laboratory assessments. Bone density measurements were carried out in a subgroup of patients who received buserelin therapy.

RESULTS

Two patients from each therapeutic group withdrew during the treatment period, for reasons unrelated to drug tolerance. Profound and consistent suppression of serial serum oestradiol-17β concentrations, to postmenopausal levels, was observed in patients receiving buserelin, while those on danazol achieved less consistent, and dose related, hypo-oestrogenism to or below early follicular phase levels.

Laparoscopic comparisons are shown in Table 1. At the post-treatment laparoscopy the mean A.F.S. score for endometriotic lesions alone was reduced from the mean score at pretreatment laparoscopy, by 86% in the buserelin group (n=38) and by 67% in the danazol group (n=18). These reductions in score were comparable in patients with mild endometriosis from both groups, but in patients with moderate and severe disease the reductions in score were more marked in patients who received buserelin.

Table 1. Laparoscopic comparisons

	Buserelin	Danazol
Total Number	38	18
Revised A.F.S. Staging:		
Mild	21	13
Moderate	10	3
Severe	7	2
Resolution of Endometriotic Lesions:		
Complete Resolution	31 (82 %)	11 (61 %)
Partial Resolution	7 (18 %)	5 (28 %)
No Change	-	2 (11 %)
Worsened	-	-

Both drugs were comparable in their efficacy in improving the subjective symptoms of dysmenorrhoea, pelvic pain and deep dsypareunia (Table 2). Although the side effects of danazol

Table 2. Side Effects

	Buserelin (n = 39) %	Danazol (n = 18) %
Hot flushes	74	22
Vaginal dryness	23	5.5
Headaches	20	39
Recurrent breakthrough bleeding	23	55
Breast size reduction	2.6	5.5
Fluid retention symptoms	8	94
Irritability/mood swings/ depression/emotional lability	10	83
Prolonged fatigue/lethargy	2.6	72
Weight gain >3 kg	-	72
Acen/seborrhoea	-	55
Hirsutism	-	22

tended to be more troublesome, and 18% of the patients on buserelin experienced severe hot flushes, none of the patients had dropped out because of these side effects. Some of the patients on buserelin have reported increased sense of well-being (14%), improved libido (8%) and the abolition of or improvement in symptoms of the premenstrual syndrome (23%). Following completion of treatment menses returned within a mean of 44 days (range 24-79) in the buserelin subjects, and 35 days (range 22-95) in the danazol patients.

A subgroup of thirteen patients treated with buserelin have been evaluated for any change in bone density which might have resulted from hypo-oestrogenism [5]. There was a significant reduction of 5.9% ($p<0.001$) in their mean lumbar vertebral trabecular bone density, as measured by quantitative computed tomography, at the end of treatment. There was also a marginally significant reduction in the mean cortical bone mineral content of 0.9% ($p=0.07$), as measured by dual photon densitometry in the right femur midshaft. Six months following discontinuation of buserelin treatment all of the lost trabecular and cortical bone had been regained.

At twelve months after discontinuation of treatment, there were 7 patients who conceived out of 11 patients from the buserelin group presenting with infertility, and 5 patients who conceived out of 10 patients in the danazol group. Recurrence of endometriosis, as diagnosed by laparoscopy, within twelve months after completion of treatment has been observed in 6 patients from the buserelin group and in 3 patients from the danazol group.

CONCLUSIONS

Both buserelin and danazol were effective in inducing a reversible state of hypo-oestrogenism, although this was more marked and consistent in patients on buserelin. While both treatments were highly effective in inducing complete or partial resolution of the endometriotic lesions, buserelin seemed more effective in patients with more severe disease. In association with this objective regression of endometriotic implants, there was a marked improvement in the subjective symptoms of endometriosis, which was comparable with both treatments. Where the two drugs differed largely was in the incidence and nature of side effects; anabolic, psychological and androgenic side effects were more predominant in the danazol treated patients, while the more tolerable vasomotor side effects predominated in the buserelin group. Pregnancy and recurrence rates were similar following both treatments. The reversible reduction in bone mass in patients receiving GnRH agonists is of major concern and needs to be further clarified.

We conclude that buserelin administered by the intranasal route offers an effective alternative to danazol in the medical management of endometriosis.

ACKNOWLEDGEMENTS

We thank Dr. Tim Spirou and Dr. Charles Matthijssen of Hoechst-Roussel, U.S.A., for support of W.H.M. on a research grant; and Dr. Patrick Magill of Hoechst, U.K., for supplying buserelin.

REFERENCES

1. Barbieri, RL, Evans, S and Kistner, RW (1982). Danazol in the treatment of endometriosis: analysis of 100 cases with a 4-year follow-up. Fertil Steril, 37, 737
2. Lemay, A, Maheux, R, Faure, N, Jean, C and Fazekas, ATA (1984). Reversible hypogonadism induced by a luteinizing hormone-releasing hormone (LHRH) agonist (Buserelin) as a new therapeutic approach for endometriosis. Fertil Steril, 41, 863
3. Shaw, RW and Matta, WHM (1986). Reversible pituitary ovarian suppression induced by an LHRH agonist in the treatment of endometriosis - comparison of two dose regimens. Clin Reprod Fertil, 4, 329
4. Revised American Fertility Society Classification of Endometriosis (1985). Fertil Steril, 43, 351
5. Matta, WHM, Shaw, RW, Hesp, R and Katz, D (1987). Hypogonadism induced by luteinising hormone releasing hormone agonist analogues: effects of bone density in premenopausal women. Brit Med J, 294, 1523

6
MANAGEMENT OF PELVIC ENDOMETRIOSIS WITH A GnRH ANALOGUE

Dominic F.H. LI and P.C. HO
Department of Obstetrics and Gynaecology
University of Hong Kong, Hong Kong

INTRODUCTION

Pelvic endometriosis remains a difficult gynaecological problem to manage and yet the progression of the disease can be very detrimental to the health of the patients. Surgical treatment often involves removal of the reproductive as well as the hormonal functions of the patient. With the discovery of GnRH analogues ability to induce reversible suppression of the hypothalamic-pituitary-ovarian axis, it becomes possible to produce a hypoestrogenic state which allows regression of the disease. This paper reports on a Phase III clinical trial on the use of buserelin (Hoechst China Ltd) in the management of patients with severe pelvic endometriosis.

METHOD

Patients between the age of 20-40 years old with moderate to severe endometriosis proven by laparoscopy or laparotomy were included in the study. Exclusion criteria included previous treatment with Danazol within the last six months, known history of allergy to GnRH analogues and patients with severe medical or endocrine diseases. After careful explanation, informed consent was obtained before the commencement of treatment. All patients were given a practicing kit with no active ingredients for intranasal spray applications, before treatment was started on the first day of the subsequent cycle after the laparoscopy or laparotomy. Buserelin 900mcg was given intranasally in three divided doses each day for six months continuously. Patients were followed up weekly for the first month, then monthly for the rest of the treatment period. Repeat laparoscopy was performed on all patients at the completion of treatment to assess the efficacy of buserelin treatment. These patients were then followed up monthly to detect for recurrence of symptoms of endometriosis.

Baseline investigations at the begining of treatment included complete blood count, liver and renal function tests, lipid profiles, serum calcium and phosphate levels. The body weight and blood pressure were also recorded. These investigations were repeated at the completion of treatment at six months. Hormonal profiles (plasma LH, FSH, E2, Progesterone, morning cortisol and serum beta-HCG) were checked at baseline, 2nd week and then monthly during the treatment and follow up period. All patients kept a diary to record any deviation of dosages or occurrence of vaginal bleeding. Any side effects arising from the treatment were recorded and symptoms of hypoestrogenism such as hot flushes and vaginal dryness were specially sought for during the follow up visits.

RESULTS

Sixteen patients were recruited into the study with mean age 34.3 ± 3.5 years old. The mean height was 156.1 ± 5.1cm and pretreatment weight was 52.7 ± 6.6kg. All patients had moderate to severe pelvic endometriosis according to the American Fertility Society (AFS) scoring system. After intranasal treatment with buserelin, 75% of patients achieved amenorrhoea within the first 5 weeks; 17% had occasional vaginal spotting and 8% had cyclical bleeding. For those with vaginal bleeding the amount was much diminished and painless. Symptoms of endometriosis were improved in all patients and totally disappeared in 63% of patients. No patient had difficulty in intranasal administration of buserelin although some might forget one or two doses because the drug was not immediately accessible (patient failure).

Side-effects of treatment were mild and uncommon: hot flushes 19%; muscle pain 19%; vaginal dryness 13%; acne 13% and nausea 6%. One patient had rather bad nausea requiring anti-emetic treatment.

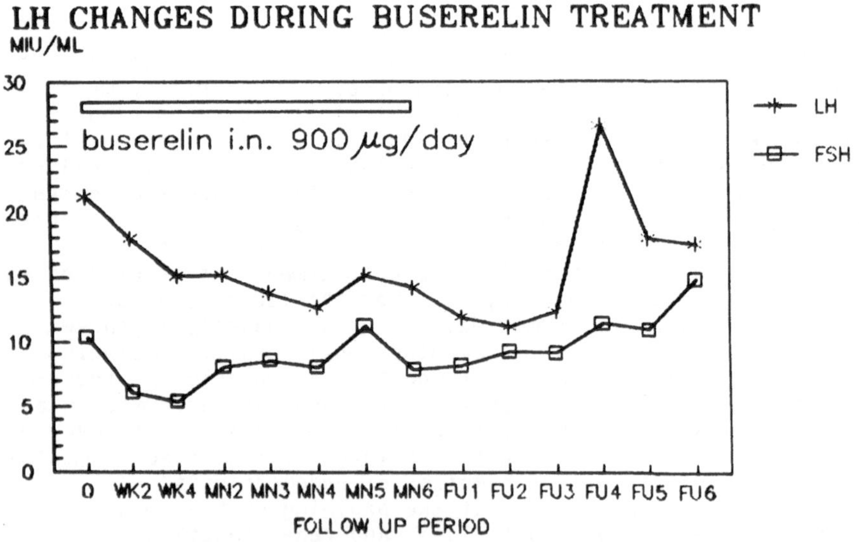

FIGURE 1 LH changes during buserelin treatment

The changes in plasma LH, FSH and estradiol during the treatment and follow up periods are shown in Figures 1 and 2. A hypogonadotrophic hypogonadal state was achieved, after a stimulatory phase at the second week of treatment Anovulation was

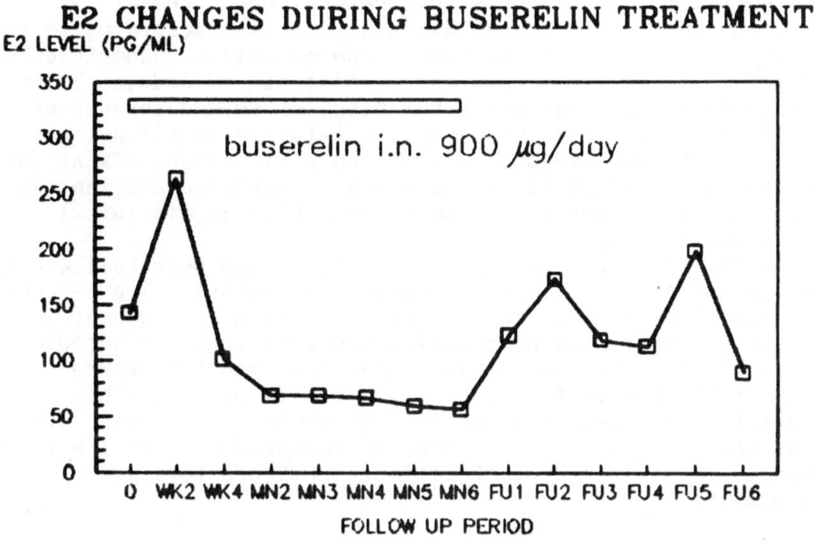

FIGURE 2 Estradiol changes during buserelin treatment

Table 1. Changes in prolactin, cortisol and lipid profiles before and after buserelin treatment. Mean (SD)

Parameter Measured	(I) Before Treatment	(II) After Treatment	(III) 6-Month Follow-up
Prolactin (ng/ml)*	14.4 (9.6)	7.8 (3.9)	10.6 (6.5)
Cortisol (mmol/l)	451 (193)	388 (144)	481 (128)
Cholesterol (mmol/l)	5.95 (5.50)	5.05 (1.04)	4.87 (1.03)
HDL-Cholesterol** (mmol/l)	1.36 (0.20)	1.57 (0.33)	1.68 (0.15)
Total Lipids (mmol/l)	5.2 (1.2)	5.5 (2.1)	5.6 (1.9)
Triglycerides (mmol/l)	2.86 (4.00)	1.77 (1.16)	1.47 (0.98)

*I vs II $p<0.03$; I vs II not significant
**I vs II $p<0.05$; I vs III $p<.001$

evident from the persistently low plasma progesterone level throughout treatment. The changes in plasma prolactin, morning cortisol and serum lipid profiles are shown in Table I. No significant changes were observed in blood counts, liver and renal function tests, serum calcium and phosphate levels.

All patients who completed treatment had a repeat laparoscopy done. All showed diminished scores according to the AFS classification of endometriosis and no active endometriosis was identified. Two patients had persistence of nodules in the rectovaginal septum clinically but biopsies showed absence of endometriotic implants. Menstruation returned in all patients after treatment was stopped: 27% at the first month; 64% at the second month and 9% at the third month. Regular ovulation was observed in all patients as evident by a rise in mid-luteal progesterone levels.

At the time of reporting, 11 patients had been followed up for a mean of 4.6 ± 1.9 months (range 2-7 months). Ten per cent of patients had moderate recurrence of symptoms of endometriosis (dysmenorrhea or rectal pain during menstruation) which could be adequately dealt with by simple analgesics (Ponston, Parke-Davis). Forty per cent of patients had mild but tolerable dysmenorrhea not requiring specific treatment. By subjective ratings the pain was much improved as compared with that before treatment. Fifty per cent of patients remained totally asymptomatic.

DISCUSSION

This study confirmed previous findings that buserelin, a GnRH analogue, causes down regulation of the GnRH receptors producing a hypogonadotrophic hypogonadal state after prolonged treatment. Effective symptomatic relief was achieved during treatment and superficial pelvic endometriosis disappeared. However, nodules in the rectovaginal septum still remained clinically palpable after treatment. These could be fibrotic nodules left behind after the endometriotic implants resorbed with buserelin treatment. Moderate symptoms reappeared in 10% of patients but the severity was much improved as evident by both subjective ratings and by the subsequent treatment required. These were the patients with cyclical spotting observed on treatment. The degree of oestrogen suppression was not complete in some cases on this standard 900 mcg/day intranasal dosage. Hence a readjustment of dosage may be required in some patients to achieve complete ovarian suppression.

As shown in other studies buserelin treatment was found to cause only mild side effects and none of the patients in this study stopped treatment because of intolerable side effects. An interesting observation in the present study was the low incidence of hot flushes in our Chinese patients as compared to other reports (19% vs 70-100%). These symptoms were specifically asked for during the follow up interview and this could not be explained by observation bias alone. In fact, hot flushes are not widely observed in Chinese patients after natural menopause either.

In conclusion, buserelin treatment was found to be effective in treatment of severe pelvic endometriosis with minor side-effects as compared with conventional medical therapy. Asymptomatic nodules within the rectovaginal septum may still be present after 6 months' therapy and long term follow up is required on these subjects to detect recurrences. Furthermore, long term safety of this form of therapy on bone and calcium metabolism needs to be documented by large scale studies.

ACKNOWLEDGEMENT

We wish to thank Hoechst China Ltd, Hong Kong to supplying the buserelin for this trial.

7
THE USE OF GnRH ANALOGUES TO CONTROL MENSTRUAL BLEEDING

R.W. SHAW
Academic Department of Obstetrics and Gynaecology,
Royal Free Hospital School of Medicine,
Pond Street, London NW3, UK

INTRODUCTION

A substantial proportion of General Practitioner consultations and gynaecological referrals concern disorders of menstrual bleeding. In the last decade an increased understanding of the mechanisms which initiate and regulate menstrual blood flow have resulted in new approaches to endeavour to control excessive or disordered menstrual bleeding.

CONTROL OF NORMAL MENSTRUAL BLEEDING

The average blood loss is about 30ml per month with a cycle between 21 and 35 days. Evaluation of menstrual blood loss poses problems for gynaecologists. Methods of assessing the number of menstrual pads used, duration of blood loss and inconvenience caused to the patient are used but show poor correlation to actual measured blood losses.

The basic understanding of morphological events in endometrial sequestration came from the classic observation studies of intra-ocular endometrial transplants in the monkey [1]. The initial change in the process of menstruation is intense arteriolar vaso-constriction in the spiral vessels, which precedes the onset of menstrual bleeding by a few hours. This vaso-constriction causes distal ischaemia with eruption of blood into the vessel wall when the vessel subsequently dilates. The process is mediated by withdrawal of ovarian steroid hormones from decreasing luteal function in the absence of pregnancy. Menstrual fluid was shown to contain vasoconstrictor agents [2] and these have subsequently been identified as prostaglandins (PG) $F_{2\alpha}$ and PGE_2. PG's action on smooth muscle is to initiate vaso-constriction of arterioles and thus PG's are the main regulating mechanism for the volume of blood that is lost at menstruation [3].

The endometrium has the capacity to synthesize PGs from exogenous arachidonic acid and prostaglandin $F_{2\alpha}$ synthesized in the endometrium stimulates vasoconstriction. PGE_2 induces modest vasodilatation of the microvasculature and PGE_2 is produced in increased amounts in the endometrium of patients with excessive menstrual losses (menorrhagia) [4]. The same authors show a significant inverse correlation between the relation of $PGF_{2\alpha}$ to PGE_2 and blood loss.

Although patients with bleeding disorders, e.g. Von Willebrands Disease and thrombocytopaenia, have increased menstrual bleeding, haemostatic mechanisms play a small role in controlling menstrual blood loss. Platelet plugs form in the vessel only during the first 24 hours of menstruation and fibrin is only detected in small amounts during the first 48 hours. However, platelets metabolise arachidonic acid to thromboxane A_2, itself a potent vasoconstrictor and platelet aggregator [5]. This demonstrates a common link between haemostatic and vaso-constrictor elements in the control of menstrual blood loss and changes that occur in dysfunctional uterine bleeding.

Detailed studies have been undertaken and have established changes in the normal mechanisms which control menstrual blood loss in patients with dysfunctional uterine bleeding and menorrhagia. There is rarely a disorder of ovarian steroidogenesis in these patients, except in adolescence and peri-menopausal patients. However, there is increased evidence for the role of eicosanoid dysfunction in this condition. Levels of both $PGF_{2\alpha}$ and E_2 are elevated within the endometrium of women with menorrhagia and such endometrium has a greater capacity to synthesise these prostaglandins [4]. Thus one of the main mechanisms contributing to dysfunctional uterine bleeding is altered prostaglandin and eicosanoid secretion and function.

DRUG THERAPY FOR MENORRHAGIA

Treatments which affect prostaglandin synthesis, fibrinolysis or have an effect on ovarian steroidogenesis are all currently utilised in efforts to control excessive menstrual bleeding. The drugs used are as listed in Table 1. Many of these agents have beneficial effects but their side-effect profiles limited their use in terms of duration or age range. Hysterectomy may be the ultimate solution but in patients still wishing to conserve their reproductive function, conservative approaches are necessary.

EFFECT OF AGONISTIC ANALOGUES OF LHRH

The normal menstrual cycle depends upon the pulsatile release of LHRH from the hypothalamus inducing pulsatile gonadotrophin release and ovarian steroidogenesis. Progressive disorders of LHRH secretion are manifested as progressive disorders of menstruation, in the most severe form as amenorrhoea. The daily administration of LHRH agonistic analogues throughout the menstrual cycle in monkeys and women results in suppression of the pituitary-ovarian axis and inhibition of ovulation [6-8]. The

TABLE 1: Medical treatments used in dysfunctional uterine bleeding

Fibrinolytic inhibitors	-	Epsilon caproic acid Transexamic acid
Altered capillary fragility	-	Ethamsylate
Prostaglandin synthetase inhibitors	-	Mefanamic acid Indomethacin Ibuprofen Naproxyn
Progestogen replacement	-	Norethisterone acetate Duphaston
Ovulation inhibition	-	Combined oral contraceptives Danazol

appreciation of this action of these agents has opened up the way for attempts to investigate their application in controlling excessive menstruation.

ADMINISTRATION OF LHRH ANALOGUES IN THE EARLY FOLLICULAR OR LUTEAL PHASE

Administration of LHRH analogues in the early follicular phase of the cycle (Days 1-3) results in an initial markedly increased secretion of LH and FSH levels 24-36 hours after administration. There is then a gradual fall towards baseline levels, FSH more rapidly than LH, with suppressed levels by the 7th and 10th days of analogue administration, respectively. This initial gonadotrophin surge prior to pituitary desensitization initiates follicular growth and oestradiol 17β elevation which then follow a similar downward trend as gonadotrophin levels. Commonly oestrogen withdrawal bleeds occur some 11-16 days after commencement of treatment at a time when oestradiol 17β levels invariably return to menstrual values. Continued administration of analogues produces suppression of LH pulsatile release, inhibition of ovulation and suppression of progesterone secretion [7, 8]. Continued inhibition of ovarian steroid hormone output, associated with suppression of the endometrial growth, results in reduction or inhibition of further menstrual bleeding.

Commencement of analogue therapy in the luteal phase of the cycle (Day 22) produces a similar increased output of gonadotrophins with a resultant accompanying increased oestradiol and progesterone secretion. This increased corpus luteal steroidogenic function results in a delay in the expected onset of menstruation of between 3 and 8 days in these patients. Menstruation commences when pituitary desensitization has occurred and ovarian steroidal hormone levels have fallen to menstrual phase values.

POSSIBLE DIRECT ANTI-OESTROGENIC ACTIONS OF LHRH ANALOGUES

The normal stimulatory action of oestrogen on the rat uterus can be inhibited by the concurrent administration of LHRH analogues [9]. It was observed that marked reduction in uterine size occurred in a group of stumptailed macaques treated with buserelin in a pilot study to control menstrual blood loss [10]. In the human female a number of patients receiving buserelin for contraceptive purposes, despite high oestrogen/progesterone ratios in the blood, had endometrial biopsies which failed to demonstrate any endometrial hyperplasia and indeed the majority of these patients had atrophic/poorly developed proliferative endometrium [11]. Exogenous progesterone injections have also failed to induce menstrual bleeding in such patients with inadequate suppression of oestradiol 17ß. These actions suggest direct blockade of LHRH analogues on the action of oestrogen and progesterone within the mymoetrium and endometrium itself, which may be of value in patients with disorders of menstrual bleeding.

EFFORTS TO CONTROL EXCESSIVE MENSTRUAL BLEEDING BY ADMINISTRATION OF LHRH ANALOGUES - ANIMAL DATA

The finding of a number of stumptailed macaques with excessive days of menstrual bleeding who had undergone many years of study in the animal colony, prompted initial study of LHRH analogues to control dysfunctional uterine bleeding. Average days of bleeding per month in these particular animals ranged between 7.5 and 15.4 days compared with a mean of 2.9 +/-0.8 in other animals in the colony. Daily vaginal swabs were taken from each animal and femoral venopunctures were made three times per week for a control period of six months prior to the administration subcutaneously daily of buserelin, 2 animals 50μg daily for a period of 5 weeks, the dose then being reduced to 10μg, and 3 animals a 10μg daily dose was given throughout. In 1 animal after 4 months treatment and failure to control bleeding, the dose was increased to 50μg daily.

The treatment with buserelin was successful in all animals to suppress steroidogenesis and inhibit ovulation. During the first treatment cycle all animals bled for about their usual duration, but in succeeding cycles 4 of the 5 animals showed consistent reduction in the number of days of bleeding with only occasional irregular losses occurring per 4 week period. One animal despite increasing the dose to 50μg daily, and despite further suppression of ovarian steroids, still continued to have eratic breakthough bleeding [10]. This study indicated that suppression of ovarian function by means of chronic LHRH agonist treatment in animals with excessive menstrual bleeding, could result in good control and warranted further studies in human subjects.

EFFECT OF LHRH AGONIST ADMINISTRATION IN WOMEN WITH DYSFUNCTIONAL UTERINE BLEEDING

The administration of buserelin, intranasally, once daily to suppress ovulation for contraceptive purposes has resulted in complete amenorrhoea in one third of subjects during treatment while the remaining two thirds had a reduced number of days of bleeding though often at irregular intervals [7, 8]. Failure of complete control of menstrual losses may be related both to the dose of LHRH analogue given and the frequency of administration and it may be necessary to give more than once daily to achieve consistent suppression of the hypothalamic-pituitary-ovarian (HPO) axis.

Initial studies in women with menorrhagia were performed on a group of women who had undergone diagnostic curettage examination to exclude pelvic pathology. At review several months later they still complained of menorrhagia and measurement of menstrual blood loss exceeded 80ml/cycle as analysed using an alkaline haematin dilution method [12]. Buserelin was then administered intranasally commencing on Day 4 following onset of menstruation. One subject had a single daily dose of 400µg and the other three subjects were given 200µg T.D.S. because of the response observed in the first patient. Treatment was continued for a period of 12 weeks during which all menstrual blood losses were measured and the number of days of bleeding recorded. In addition, 3 times per week early morning urine samples were collected and analysed for oestrogen/ creatinine and pregnanediol/creatinine. Following cessation of treatment all menstrual pads were collected for a further two spontaneous menstrual cycles.

Menstrual losses in these subjects ranged between 95 and 198ml/month. Following treatment in all subjects, blood loss was reduced during the treatment phase and it became apparent during the second and third treatment months that blood loss was reduced to between 0 and 30ml/month. During the first cycle of treatment a slight increase in ovarian oestrogen secretion in the first 2-3 weeks of therapy was observed, but despite this 3 of the 4 patients had fewer days of bleeding than their normal cycle, though one patient, on the single daily dosage of buserelin, had eratic spotting for much of the first cycle.

Failing to give a large enough dose of buserelin to induce sufficient inhibition of ovarian steroidogenesis resulted in one patient being converted from ovulatory cycles to anovulatory cycles with quite marked oestrogen stimulation and persistent bleeding. With a larger increased dose of buserelin and three times per day application, this feature was not observed in the remaining three patients, all of whom had quite low oestrogen/creatinine levels throughout therapy (see Fig. 1).

Overall the therapy was extremely successful in reducing measured menstrual blood loss as shown in Table 2. Following

TABLE 2: Measured menstrual blood losses (ml/4 weeks) in subjects with menorrhagia receiving buserelin 200 ug T.D.S. intranasally.

	PRE-TREATMENT		TREATMENT MONTHS			POST-TREATMENT MONTHS	
Patient	1	2	1	2	3	1	2
1	94	112	90	25	15	63	88
2	162	148	24	18	Nil	45	372
3	108	98	22	Nil	Nil	65	102
4*	143	186	41	32	28	94	N/A

*400 ug once daily in subject 4; N/A - No assay available.

cessation of therapy with buserelin, the first spontaneous menstrual period ocurred between 16 and 27 days, and in 3 of the 4 cycles these were judged to be ovulatory (Fig. 1). With the return of ovarian function there was also an increased amount of menstrual blood loss. Patients returned towards their previous increased losses and by the second month after treatment all had exceeded 80ml/month again.

To evaluate whether even more profound suppression of the HPO axis could be achieved with better control of excessive menstrual loss, we studied the effect of a depot LHRH preparation, goserelin (Zoladex® ICI Pharmaceuticals), which contains 3.6mg of LHRH analogue in a 50:50 lactic/glycolic acid co-polymer depot, which is designed to release drug continuously over 28 days. In this study a group of patients with menorrhagia with measured blood loss in excess of 80ml/month were evaluated in a pre-treatment phase as above and then given 3 single goserelin depots at 4 weekly intervals for a treatment period of 12 weeks. The first depot was inserted on Day 2-3 of the menstrual cycle. All blood losses were measured during the treatment phase and during the two cycles following the last depot. Table 3 indicates

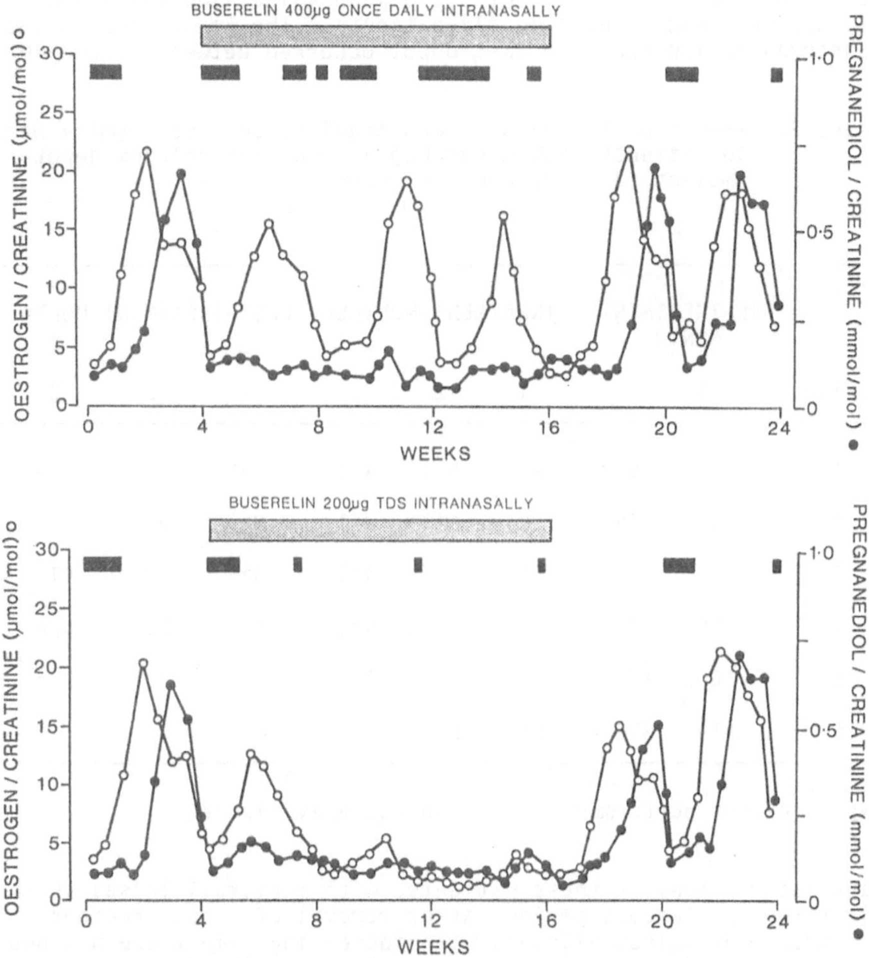

FIGURE 1 Patterns of urinary oestrogen/creatinine and urinary pregnanediol/creatinine ratio in two patients receiving Buserelin. Patient receing 400µg once daily had conversion from ovulatory to anovulatory cycles. Patient receiving 200µg t.d.s. had adequate suppression and control of menstrual losses

that blood loss was reduced in all 6 patients quite dramatically. Two experienced no bleeding whatsoever following the first implant despite the expected initial agonist induced stimulatory rise of gonadotrophins and oestradiol-17β. Only one of the six patients had further bleeding episodes following administration of the 2nd and 3rd implants at 4 and 8 weeks. The circulating oestradiol 17β was suppressed in all patients to a mean value <100pmol/l and hot flushes were experienced by all patients. The first spontaneous menstrual period from the last depot occurred between 56 and 70

TABLE 3: Reduction in measured menstrual blood losses (ml/4 weeks) in patients with menorrhagia receiving zoladex depot implant (3.6 mg) every 4 weeks.

	PRE-TREATMENT MONTH		TREATMENT MONTHS			POST-TREATMENT MONTHS		
Patient	1	2	1	2	3	1	2	3
1	80	84	Nil	Nil	Nil	32	21	N/A
2	112	99	53	Nil	Nil	Nil	68	51
3	102	81	54	Nil	Nil	Nil	18	41
4	98	84	51	Nil	Nil	41	39	N/A
5	160	107	50	41	32	61	72	N/A
6	419	370	Nil	Nil	Nil	*		

*Hysterectomy performed. N/A = no assay available.

days later. None of these patients, with menstrual losses in the first two spontaneous periods after removal of depot, reached pre-treatment values although with increasing time there has been a return towards excessive menstrual losses. The study further confirms the effective inhibition of excessive bleeding by the use of LHRH analogues, but perhaps points to more effective suppression when depot preparations are utilized. The depot preparations also seem to result in a prolonged period before return to normal menstrual losses and this may reflect qualitative alteration in gonadotrophin secretion that has not been studied in detail in our own patients.

MENORRHAGIA IN ASSOCIATION WITH UTERINE FIBROIDS

A frequent accompanying symptom of uterine fibroids is menorrhagia. Our initial pilot animal study [10] suggested that when uterine fibroids were present there may be less reduction in menstrual loss by LHRH analogues. To study this we have monitored menstrual bleeding in a group of women receiving nafarelin (Synarel®, Syntex Pharmaceuticals) 250μg daily intranasally for treatment of uterine fibroids with mean size equivalent of 14.8 weeks pregnancy, who also complained of menorrhagia. The total blood losses were not measured but pre-treatment days of menstruation were a mean of 7.4 +/- 1.8 days. Six of the 11 patients had haemoglobin values less than 10.4g/dl on admission to the study. Patients received the nafarelin treatment for a period of 6 months and recorded the number of days of menstrual bleeding in each four week cycle. This was compared with an age matched group of patients receiving nafarelin 250μg twice daily as treatment for endometriosis over a six months period, and who recorded the number of days of menstrual bleeding in a comparable manner. Hormonal assays confirmed that the degree of oestrogen suppression achieved in the two groups of patients was similar with serum oestradiol 17β values of 112 +/- 10.8 pmol/l and 88.4 +/- 8.3 pmol/l at 3 and 6 months treatment respectively in the uterine fibroid group and at comparable times with values of 106 +/- 11.4 pmol/l in the endometriosis group of patients. Bleeding patterns of the two groups of patients are shown in Table 4 and 5.

TABLE 4: Effect of administering nafarelin 250 ug twice daily intranasally on number of days of menstrual bleeding experienced by women with fibroids.

Month	DAYS OF MENSTRUAL BLEEDING PER PATIENT										
	1	2	3	4	5	6	7	8	9	10	11
1	8	6	18	9	11	2	8	10	13	14	10
2	1					9	11	10	17	10	13
3							8	10	9	1	22
4								9	18	3	9
5								12	22	1	4
6								15	17	1	2

All patients experienced bleeding within the first cycle of nafarelin administration and in each of the 11 subjects with fibroids and menorrhagia this was greater than their normal average loss in terms of days, but less in perceived amount and in 6 of the 11 patients in the endometriosis group this same finding was observed. However, following this first month of treatment a marked difference was seen between patients with menorrhagia and fibroids and those with endometriosis in the bleeding episodes, there clearly being more days of bleeding in patients with fibroids and indeed 4 patients bled each cycle during the 6 months

TABLE 5: Effect of administering nafarelin 250 ug twice daily intranasally on number of days of menstrual bleeding experienced by women with endometriosis.

Month	DAYS OF MENSTRUAL BLEEDING PER PATIENT									
	1	2	3	4	5	6	7	8	9	10
1	5	13	15	14	6	5	15	8	15	7
2								4	3	3
3									-	2
4									3	
5									-	
6									5	

of treatment on many days, whilst this was only seen in one patient undergoing treatment for endometriosis. Further studies are therefore required in menorrhagia associated with uterine fibroids to determine whether despite a marked degree of HPO suppression, control of menstrual bleeding may not be as effective. This may reflect a fundamental difference in the causes of menorrhagia between subjects with fibroids and those with dysfunctional uterine bleeding, and denote a need to obtain greater HPO axis suppression.

SUMMARY

Despite quite a number and range of medical therapies being available to control menorrhagia, few have effects which persist after treatment. This suggests that current treatments do not correct the underlying pathology which, in the majority of patients with dysfunctional uterine bleeding, is one of altered prostaglandin/prostacyclin production and/or sensitivity.

Studies reported here indicate that LHRH analogues offer an alternative and successful therapeutic approach and should be able to control quite efficiently and quickly menstrual blood loss in patients with menorrhagia. However, sustained hypo-oestrogenism to within the menopausal range may be necessary to achieve consistent control of blood loss and this could induce changes in bone calcium homeostasis with increased calcium excretion and reduction of bone mineral content [14]. The role of LHRH analogue therapy in dysfunctional uterine bleeding and excessive menstrual blood loss in patients with fibroids, seems to be limited to a short duration of application, perhaps between 6 and 12 months but perhaps has its greatest role to play in its use for a period of 4-6 months prior to surgery to facilitate that surgery. Recent work indicates that administration of LHRH analogues reduces the uterine size and alters the arterial blood flow as measured by the Resistant Index using Doppler ultrasound . This suggests a marked and significant reduction in blood flow following 4 months of LHRH agonist administration [15].

The thoughts that these analogues may be beneficial in patients in the peri-menopausal period to tide them through to the menopause, however, need to be tempered in view of the effects on mineral bone content. Any increased bone loss occurring during the analogue therapy will only complement that expected during the early post-menopausal period.

ACKNOWLEDGEMENTS

My thanks to Dr. Rosemary Gardner for menstrual loss measurements and to Hoechst Pharmaceuticals, Syntex Pharmaceuticals and I.C.I. Pharmaceuticals for supplies of LHRH analogues used in these studies.

REFERENCES

1. Markee, JE (1940). Menstruation in intraocular endometrial transplants in the rhesus monkey. Contr Embryol Carn Ins, 28, 219
2. Pickles, VR, and Hall, WJ (1963). Some physiological properties of the menstrual stimulant substances A1 and A2. J Reprod Fertil, 6, 315
3. Abel, M (1979). Production of prostaglandins by the human uterus: are they involved in menstruation? Res Clinic Forums, 1, 33
4. Smith, SK, Abel, MH, Kelly, RW, and Baird, DT (1981). Prostaglandin synthesis in the endometrium of women with ovular dysfunctional uterine bleeding. Brit J Obstet Gynaecol, 88, 434
5. Hamberg, M, and Samuellsson B (1974). Prostaglandin endoperoxides. Novel transformations of arachidonic acid in human platelets. Proc Natl Acad Sci USA, 71, 3400
6. Fraser, HM, Laird, NC, and Blakeley, DM (1980). Decreased pituitary responsiveness and inhibition of the luteinizing hormone surge and ovulation in the stumptailed monkey (Macaca arrctoides) by chronic treatment with an agonist of luteinizing hormone-releasing hormone. Endocrinology, 115, 1780
7. Bergquist, C, Nillius, SJ, and Wide, L (1982). Long-term intranasal luteinizing hormone-releasing hormone agonist treatment for contraception in women. Fertil Steril, 38, 190

8. Schmidt-Gollwitzer, M, Hardt, W, Schmidt-Gollwitzer, K, Von der Ohne, M, and Nevinny-Stickel, J (1981). Influence of the LH-RH analogue buserelin on cyclic ovarian function and on endometrium. A new approach to fertility control? Contraception, 23, 187
9. Pedroza E, Vilchez-Martinez, JA, Coy, DH, Arimura, A, and Schally, AV (1978). Correlation between in vivo inhibition of gonadotrophin release induced by LHRH and the blockade of ovulation by synthetic analogues of LHRH. Int J Fertil, 23, 294
10. Fraser, HM, and Shaw, RW (1984). Effects of chronic luteinizing hormone-releasing hormone agonist treatment in dysfunctional uterine bleeding in the stumptailed macaque. Acta Endocrinol, 106, 381
11. Bergquist, C, Nillius, SJ, Wide, L, and Lindgren, A (1981). Endometrial patterns in women on chronic luteinizing hormone-releasing hormone agonist treatment for contraception. Fertil Steril, 36, 339
12. Hallberg, L, and Nilsson, L (1964). Determination of menstrual blood loss. Scand J Clin Lab Invest, 16, 244
13. Shaw, RW, Fraser, HM, and Boyle, H (1983). Intranasal LHRH agonist treatment in women with endometriosis. Brit Med J, 287, 1667
14. Matta, WH, Shaw, RW, Hesp, R, and Katz, D (1987). Hypogonadism induced by luteinizing hormone releasing hormone agonist analogues: effects on bone density in pre-menopausal women. Brit Med J, 294, 1523
15. Matta, WH, Stabile, I, Shaw, RW, and Campbell, S (1988). Doppler assessment of uterine blood flow changes in patients with fibroids receiving the gonadotrophin-releasing hormone agonist buserelin. Fertil Steril (in press)

8

RATIONALE, INDICATIONS AND MANAGEMENT OF GnRH ANALOGUES IN OVULATION INDUCTION PROTOCOLS

B. LUNENFELD*, V. INSLER, E. LUNENFELD**, G. POTASHNIK**, and J. LEVY****

*Institute of Endocrinology, Sheba Medical Center and Bar-Ilan University, Ramat Gan, Israel

**Division of Obstetrics and Gynecology, Soroka Medical Center and Ben-Gurion University of the Negev, Beer-Sheba, Israel

INTRODUCTION

The ovulatory cycle is governed and accompanied by characteristic protein and steroid hormonal levels that are reflected by typical changes in the reproductive organs. To enable grouping, superimposition, recording and comparison of various parameters of the ovulatory cycle, to define and characterize abnormalities and to plan rational therapeutic approaches, its span is divided into several phases. Each phase reflects a characteristic, easily definable hormonal or organic change. Depending on the criteria on which the division is based, several different phases of the ovulatory cycle may be recognized. In the following discussion the simple division into follicular, ovulatory and luteal phases will be used.

The follicular phase actually begins 4-5 days before menstrual bleeding and lasts until the appearance of the LH surge. It encompasses the periods of follicular recruitment, selection of the dominant follicle, its development, growth and maturation. It is characterized by elevated levels of FSH and low levels of LH, estrogens and progesterone during the recruitment and selection phases. This is followed by an increase of estrogens during the development, growth and maturation of the dominant follicle.

The ovulatory phase is characterized by the estrogen evoked LH surge, followed by a decline in estrogen levels and a rise in progesterone levels. This is accompanied by the resumption of the first meiotic division of the oocyte, rupture of the follicle and extrusion of the egg.

The post ovulatory or luteal phase is characterized by a marked rise in progesterone levels, which reach a plateau about five days after ovulation. Concomitant with the rise in progesterone levels, the basal body temperature (BBT) increases. The association of estrogen and progesterone prepares the uterus for implantation of the fertilized egg and inhibits FSH and LH secretion via the negative feedback control at the hypothalamic and pituitary level. FSH and LH remain low during the luteal phase.

If ovulation is followed by fertilization and conception, than by the ninth post ovulatory day hCG appears in the circulation. Its rapid rise stimulates corpus luteum function expressed by a further increase in both estrogens and progesterone. In the absence of conception the corpus luteum regresses and estrogen and progesterone levels decline around the tenth day following ovulation. This marks the beginning of the late luteal (premenstrual) phase. The declining levels of estrogens and progesterone cause endometrial shedding (menstruation) and provoke the increase of FSH which marks the beginning of follicular recruitment of the following cycle.

FOLLICULAR DEVELOPMENT

Early studies, based on animal experiments, suggested that follicular development up to the antrum stage was gonadotropin independent [1, 2]. Lunenfeld and Eshkol [3] showed that in gonadotropin deprived prepubertal mice, follicular development could proceed, however it was markedly altered and retarded. It has been suggested by Gougeon [4] that in women it may take about 10 weeks for an oocyte surrounded by a single layer of granulosa cells (primordial follicle) to develop into an antral follicle capable of gonadotropic responsiveness. Final growth, maturation and ovulation will then occur within two weeks, provided that FSH and LH stimulation is adequate and the ovary is capable of a normal response.

Whereas several hundred primordial follicles probably start to grow, no more than about 20 precursor follicles are likely to be present at the beginning of the menstrual cycle [5]. All the others degenerate at early stages of development. Under physiological conditions, of the twenty remaining follicles some will be selected for further growth and development, but only one will mature, reach dominance and ovulate. The others will undergo atresia or luteinization.

According to Hodgen's group [6] in the primate model the gonadotropin dependent folliculogenesis process proceeds in the following steps:

1. **Recruitment of a follicular cohort** is dependent on rise of FSH levels which take place 4-5 days before the onset of menstrual bleeding [7, 8].
2. **Selection of a dominant follicle** from the recruited follicular cohort. This follicle is destined to reach the state of full maturity and subsequently ovulate. The selection process is completed during the early follicular phase (usually within the first seven days of the cycle).
3. **Follicular dominance**. Following its selection, the dominant follicle grows and matures at a higher rate than the other follicles, due to its increased sensitivity to FSH. Moreover, by producing estrogen as well as inhibit, the dominant follicle regulates gonadotropin secretion. This enables its final maturation and inhibits further development of other follicles of the same cohort.

4. The dominant follicle at the proper time causes the occurrence of the estrogen provoked LH surge, subsequently ovulates and is transformed into a functional corpus luteum (Fig. 1).

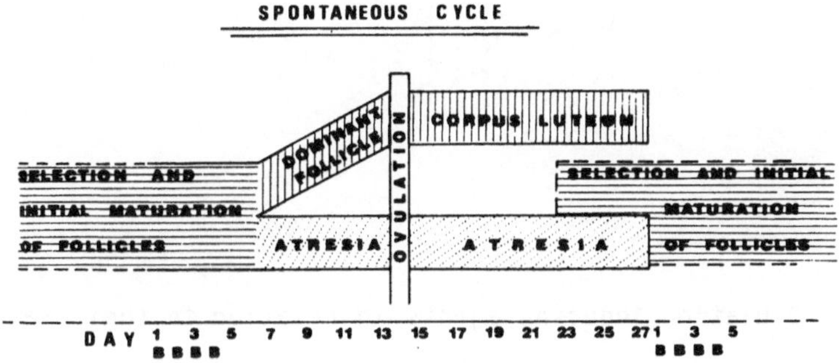

FIGURE 1 Schematic representation of different stages of a spontaneous ovulatory cycle

Any disruption in the delicately co-ordinated interaction between the integrated components of the hypothalamic-pituitary-ovarian axis (which must operate within precise quantitative limits and accurate temporal sequences) may lead to anovulation.

Disturbances in the pulsatile pattern of GnRH secretion or improper gonadotropin stimulation will derange follicular development and may result in anovulation. The severity of this situation may range from hypoestrogenic amenorrhea to regular cycles with only subtle abnormalities in follicular development and hormonal profiles in women with "unexplained infertility" [9]. The above outlined advances in reproductive endocrinology have led to a better understanding of the basic mechanisms regulating these processes and governing reproductive function. This has furnished the impetus for transforming the field of female infertility from a largely empirical approach to a more rational basis. During the last three decades a variety of effective ovulation inducing agents have been developed (Fig. 2).

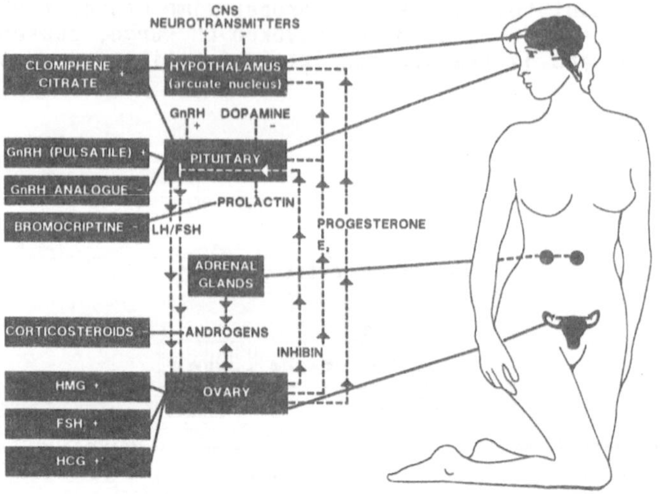

FIGURE 2 Ovulation inducing agents in relation to their targets

PRINCIPLES OF OVULATION INDUCTION

Ovulation induction necessitates FSH in the early phase of the cycle for recruitment and selection of follicles, while for growth and maturation both FSH and LH are necessary. In cases of in vitro fertilization, where the aim is to obtain multiple oocytes, increased gonadotropin stimulation should theoretically commence during the early recruitment phase, while for in vivo ovulation induction purposes, where one should aim at one or two mature follicles, gonadotropin stimulation should be delayed to the selection phase.

The basic principles of gonadotropin therapy were proposed by Insler & Lunenfeld [10, 11] following observation of the course of treatment in several hundreds of patients. Ovarian response can be elicited only when an effective daily dose of FSH-like material has been applied. Administration of gonadotropins at levels significantly below the effective daily dose does not evoke any measurable effect even when prolonged therapy is used.

Following the application of the effective daily dose of gonadotropins several ovarian follicles are stimulated to begin growth and maturation. This period of gonadotropin therapy is called the latent phase. Since at this stage of follicular development appreciable amounts of estrogen are not yet secreted and since the size of the follicles is too small to be precisely measured by ultrasound, the latent phase of therapy is clinically "mute". The latent phase begins with the application of the effective daily dose of gonadotropins and ends with the appearance of a measurable ovarian reponse, i.e. rising estrogen levels and increasing follicular diameter.

The second part of gonadotropin therapy, called the active phase lasts from the initial estrogen rise until ovulation induction. It is characterized by an exponential rise of estrogen levels and a steady growth in follicular diameter (Fig. 3).

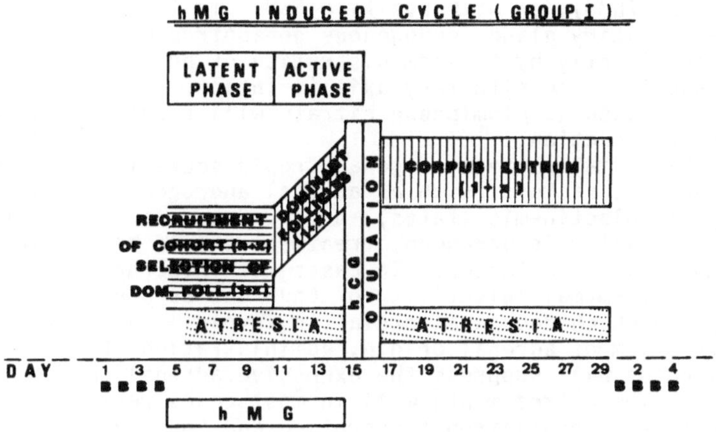

FIGURE 3 Schematic representation of different events in gonadotropin induced cycles

The above principles, based on clinical observation and a thorough analysis of patients' response, received powerful theoretical support from the experimental work of Hodgen and his group on primates [12-14].

The introduction of sonography for monitoring of follicular size and direct laparoscopy for IVF programs allowed observation of the size and appearance of ovarian follicles. This, together with the appreciation of the maturity of ova, leant further support to the empirically developed principles of gonadotropin therapy.

The latent phase of gonadotropin therapy represents a telescoping of the recruitment and selection phases of the spontaneous cycle in which the active phase of therapy corresponds to the period of dominance.

Gonadotropin therapy poses several interesting theoretical problems. The exact size of the follicular cohort recruited in each cycle in the human is not known. It is thus impossible to know whether gonadotropin therapy, using non-physiological doses, provokes the initial development of a larger cohort. Whatever the size of the initial cohort recruited, it seems that during the course of gonadotropin therapy additional follicles are stimulated and undergo partial or full maturation. Others are rescued from atresia by the sustained high level of FSH. This process results in the development of several dominant follicles that reach full maturation hours or maybe even days apart one from the other.

Enhancement of gonadotropin stimulation can be obtained by direct stimulation of the ovaries with human Menopausal Gonadotropins (hMG), or with purified FSH. In the presence of a receptive pituitary gland, endogenous gonadotropin secretion can be enhanced directly by the administration of pulsatile GnRH. When the hypothalamic-pituitary axis is intact, administration of antiestrogens such as clomiphene citrate will result in increased gonadotropin secretion.

If the normal pattern of gonadotropin secretion is disturbed by extra gonadal factors (such as adrenal androgens, peripheral fat or hyperprolactinemic states), or the frequency and amplitude of GnRH pulsatility is deranged, treatment should be oriented towards the causative factor. In cases with hyperprolactinemia restoration of normal pulsatility of GnRH can be achieved using bromocryptine which decreases prolactin levels. In cases of hyperandrogenism of adrenal origin, administration of glucocorticoids will suppress the excessive adrenal androgen production. These treatments will in most cases restore the normal pattern of gonadotropin secretion and thus result in ovulatory cycles.

In pituitary insufficiency or in cases where enhancement of endogenous gonadotropin secretion with the above mentioned agents has failed, direct stimulation with gonadotropins is indicated. However, except in cases of hypothalamic insufficiency, endogenous gonadotropins acting in concert with the hMG or FSH may interfere with the development of normal dominant follicles. If this is the case, endogenous gonadotropin secretion can be depressed by desensitization of the gonadotropes with GnRH agonist analogues. Once the cyclic pattern of endogenous gonadotropin secretion is suppressed hMG or FSH can be administered simultaneously with the analogues, to result in normal development.

Since the ovarian response to gonadotropins is dose dependent, the lowest dose which will cause orderly follicular development and function should be used for the treatment of anovulation. This can be assured by ultrasonography and estradiol measurements. Following follicular stimulation with hMG or FSH, ovulation should be induced by administration of hCG at the time when one or two follicles have reached or exceeded a diameter of 15mm and estradiol levels are between 450 and 900pg/ml. When more than two large follicles are present or when estradiol levels are excessive, hCG administration should be withheld and the treatment cycle aborted.

HYPOTHALAMIC-PITUITARY INSUFFICIENCY

Amenorrhea in women who fail to have withdrawal vaginal bleeding following progesterone challenge may be due to hypothalamic-pituitary insufficiency. Bleeding following cyclic estrogen/progesterone administration will eliminate uterine causes such as congenital abnormalities or severe uterine adhesions (Asherman's syndrome). A low or normal FSH and LH will rule out ovarian failure and point to pituitary insufficiency.

Most women with pituitary insufficiency will benefit from hMG/hCG therapy. In amenorrheic patients with hypothalamic-pituitary failure the pregnancy rate following hMG/hCG therapy is very high. In our series of 279 patients, 82% conceived [15]. This high conception rate is due to the fact that in this condition there is an absence of endogenous gonadotropin secretion. Orderly follicular development can therefore be induced with individual and well controlled administration of exogenous gonadotropins. The pituitary in these patients will not respond to the rising estrogens with a spontaneous LH surge, so that ovulation is induced with hCG when the follicles are of sufficient size and maturity.

When using human gonadotropins for induction of ovulation, one has to accept the fact that some features of the spontaneous ovulatory cycle can not be reproduced. These features are:

* Premenstrual recruitment and initial selection of follicles
* Feedback control of gonadotropin levels
* Balanced effect of intraovarian sex steroids
* Full maturation of one follicle only
* Exact synchronization of structural, functional and hormonal events throughout the entire genital system.

HYPOTHALAMIC DYSFUNCTION WITH NORMAL PROLACTIN AND ANDROGEN LEVELS

Failure to ovulate in non-androgenized normoprolactinemic women, secondary to chronic hypothalamic dysfunction, is probably the most common cause of ovulatory dysfunction. Patients in this category present with a variety of symptoms which may range from luteal phase defects to amenorrhea. This form of amenorrhea usually respond to a progesterone challenge with vaginal bleeding.

Stress, alterations in body weight, and excessive athletic activity can result in chronic hypothalamic anovulation. If change in lifestyle does not restore ovulation, clomiphene citrate is the first line therapy. The pregnancy rate following clomiphene citrate administration to 8843 normoprolactinemic patients with hypothalamic-pituitary dysfunction was only 33% despite an assumed ovulation rate of 80% [15].

The discrepancy between the ovulation rate of about 80% and the conception rate of about 33% has been attributed to abnormal tubal transport, cervical mucus hostility due to clomiphene's antiestrogenic properties, and to luteal phase inadequacy or ovum entrapment within the follicle. The latter phenomenon may be due to an untimely release of LH in response to the excess rise of estrogens, due to multiple follicular stimulation characteristic for clomiphene therapy. Treatment with hMG/hCG has been effective in about one third of patients who failed to conceive when treated with clomiphene (Fig. 4).

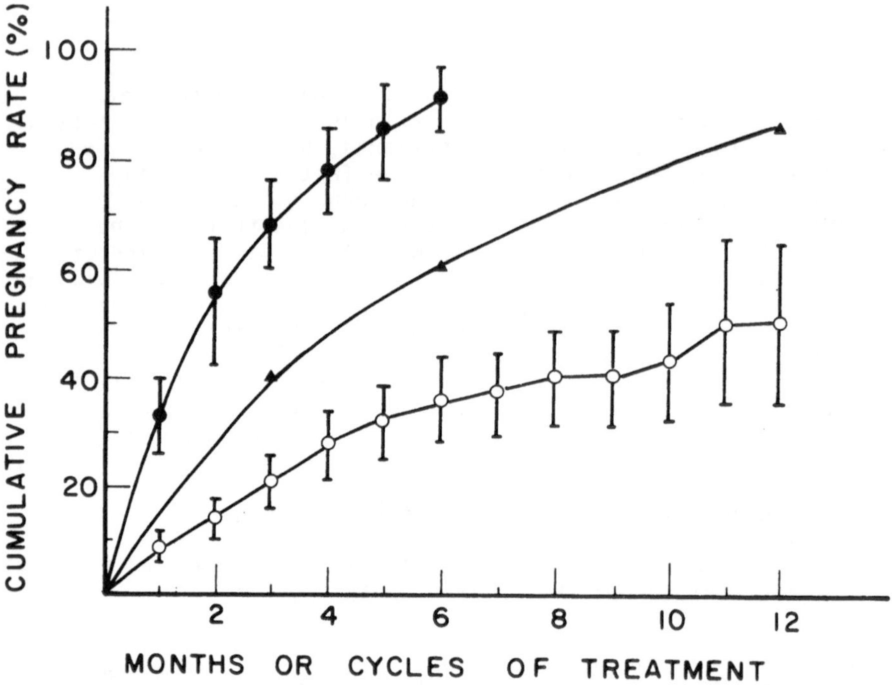

FIGURE 4 Cumulative pregnancy rates in the normal population (Δ) in women with hypothalamic-pituitary failure (o—o) and in patients with hypothalamic-pituitary dysfunction treated with clomiphene citrate (•—•)

The number of patients who have received pulsatile GnRH is still too small to permit valid conclusions. Of 155 patients given this treatment regime for 301 cycles, 61 (39%) conceived [15]. Bringer et al., [16] reviewed 439 GnRH treatment cycles which resulted in 41 conceptions (9% per cycle).

The lack of conception following these therapies may again be explained by disorderly follicular development caused by the simultaneous action of endogenous and exogenous gonadotropins. Alternatively, premature luteinization due to an untimely LH surge in response to exessive rise of estrogens may be mistaken as ovulation. The treatment of choice for such patients is a triphasic therapeutic approach. GnRH agonist is administered until the cyclic secretion pattern of endogenous gonadotropins is inhibited and the positive feedback is abolished. Thereafter hMG is given in conjunction with the GnRH agonist, in order to eliminate possible disturbing effects of the endogenous gonadotropin secretion. The rising estrogens from the follicular development will not evoke a spontaneous LH surge. When at least one follicle reaches maturation, hCG is administered to induce ovulation (Fig. 5). These previously bad responders, now

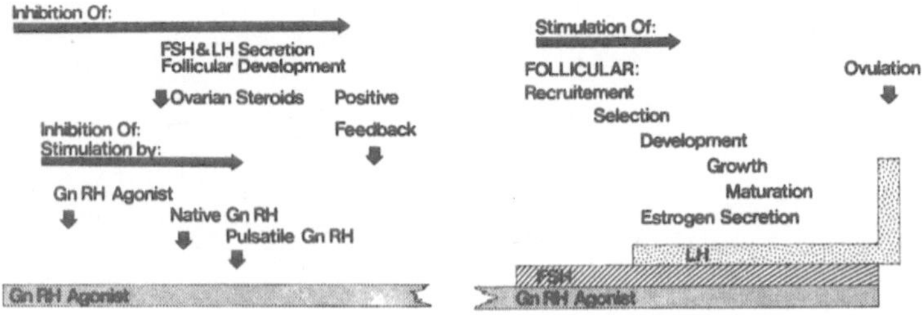

FIGURE 5 Schematic representation of the principles of triphasic therapy. Suppression of the pituitary-ovarian axis by GnRH agonist followed by concomitant gonadotropin stimulation of follicular growth and ovulation induction by hCG

converted to women with hypothalamic-pituitary insufficiency, may ovulate and conceive. Although the number of patients treated so far is still insufficient to come to statistically significant conclusions, the results seem promising.

PREMATURE LUTEINIZATION

Premature luteinization may be the cause of a specific ovulatory disturbance. This entity is frequently unrecognized or misdiagnosed as unexplained infertility, luteal phase defect, or luteinized unruptured follicle (LUF) syndrome. This situation will occur if an LH surge appears in response to rising estrogen at a time when the follicle is still immature. It can only be diagnosed if an LH peak can be detected in the presence of immature follicles as seen on ultrasonography. It may be due to an exaggerated sensitivity of the pituitary to rising estrogen. This may explain the failure of clomiphene citrate or hMG to restore ovulation in these cases. Both these agents cause multiple follicular development with exaggerated estrogen responses, thus premature LH peaks are even more likely to occur (Fig. 6). In those cases the only rational therapy is to abolish the estrogen evoked positive feedback mechanism.

This can be effectively accomplished by the use of GnRH agonists [17]. Thus, in anovulation due to recurrent premature luteinization, the treatment of choice is again the triphasic therapeutic approach (Fig. 7).

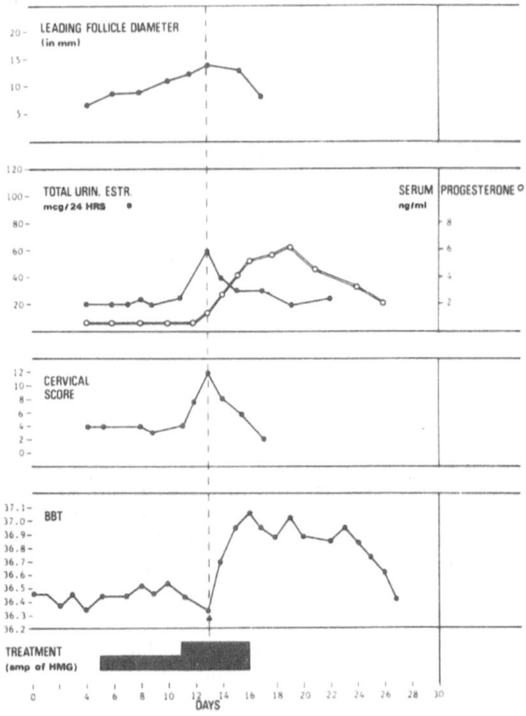

FIGURE 6 A course of gonadotropic therapy complicated by a spontaneous untimely LH surge

Our experience with the triphasic therapy produced some interesting and relevant facts which may be helpful in planning this type of treatment. Three different preparations were examined: nasal spray of [D-Ser(tBu)^{6},Pro^{9}-NHEt]LHRH (Buserelin, Hoechst, West Germany) and [D-Trp^{6}]LHRH (Decapeptyl, Ferring, West Germany) by either daily or monthly injections. Plasma FSH levels were slightly, but not significantly, elevated during the first 5 days of GnRH agonist application. From day 15 on, the FSH levels were significantly lower.

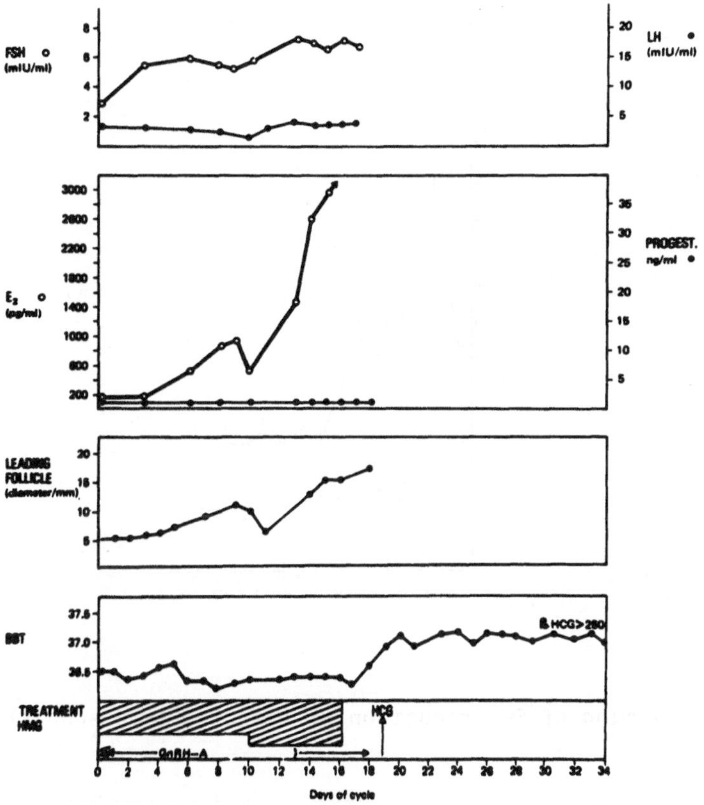

FIGURE 7 A course of gonadotropic therapy following suppression of the pituitary-ovarian axis by GnRH agonist

The levels of LH increased significantly after beginning treatment with GnRH agonists, remained high for 5 days and decreased sharply thereafter. The mean levels of LH were significantly lower on day 15 through day 28 of therapy as compared to basal levels (Fig. 9). There is a suggestion that the effect of pituitary down regulation may be particularly significant in patients with polycystic ovarian disease or in peri-menopausal women.

As judged by estradiol levels, down regulation of the pituitary-ovarian axis was achieved within 14 days in 77% and within 28 days of treatment in 95% of patients (Table 1).

FIGURE 8 Mean levels and SEM of FSH and Lh in 51 women during suppression with GnRH agonists

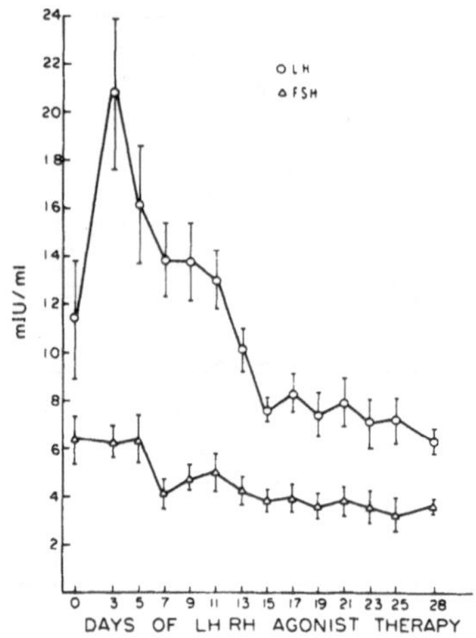

TABLE 1: Timing of E-2 reduction effected by GnRH agonists.

NO. OF DAYS OF GnRH ADMINISTRATION	NO. OF PATIENTS STUDIED	ESTRADIOL NO.	<24 PG/ML %
≤ 7	40	6	15.0
≤15	39	30	76.9
≤28	37	35	94.6

TABLE 2: Different treatment parameters in combined GnRH agonist/ gonadortopin therapy compared to treatment with gonadotropins alone in ovulation induction program.

PARAMETER	GnRH AGONIST + GONADOTROPINS MEAN	RANGE	GONADOTROPINS ALONE MEAN	RANGE
DURATION OF TREATMENT (DAYS)	16.6	3 - 28	11.1	5 - 20
TOTAL hMG DOSE (AMP)	26.4	5 - 48	16.5	5 - 34
EFFECTIVE DAILY DOSE (AMP)	1.7	1 - 3.5	1.7	1 - 3.0
LATENT PHASE (DAYS)	6.2	3 - 9	5.9	3 - 9
ACTIVE PHASE (DAYS)	6.8	3 - 9	5.1	3 - 7

As assessed by reduced levels of gonadotropins and estradiol as well as by the abolishment of the hypophyseal response to rising estrogens, down regulation of the pituitary-ovarian axis required between 14 and 21 days of GnRH agonist application. Since all the parameters were evident at approximately same time, the level of endogenous estradiol may be used as a single, sufficient indicator.

Stimulation of the ovarian function, when carried out in the presence of a suppressed pituitary-ovarian axis, required a higher dose of gonadotropins and a longer treatment time (Table 2). It also resulted in a higher number of follicles. These follicles, however, did not mature quicker or better as measured by their size or by their capacity to produce estrogens (Fig. 9). The production of fertilizable and cleavable ova was also not significantly increased. The combination of pituitary down regulation with exogenous ovarian stimulation thus appears effective but the selection of patients and the therapeutic protocols need further attention.

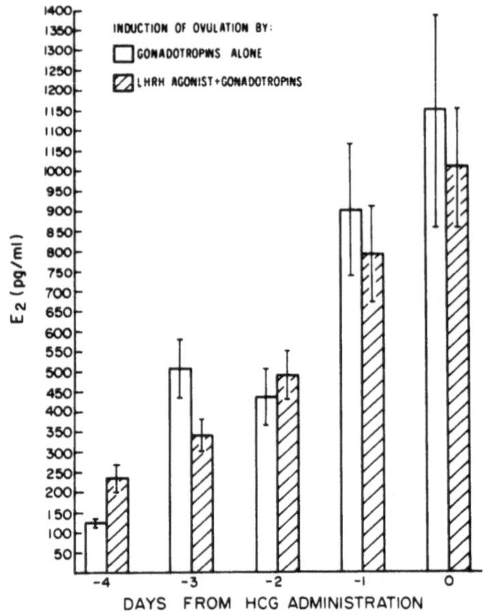

FIGURE 9 E-2 levels in patients with induction of ovulation by gonadotropins alone and by combined GnRH agonist + hMG therapy

It can be concluded that the anovulatory patient today has a 60-80% chance to take home a healthy baby. For infertility due to mechanical factors, microsurgery and IVF procedures have also improved the grim prognosis of the past. However, the chances of conception of 60-70% for tubal anastomosis or adhesiolysis, between 20-30% for neosalpingostomy and from 10-20% for IVF (18), are still significantly lower than the conception rates achievable in infertility due to various endocrine disturbances.

REFERENCES

1. Greep, RP (1963). Histology, histochemistry and ultrastructure of adult ovary. In: Grady, HG and Smith, DE (eds.) "The Ovary". p.48. (Baltimore: Williams & Wilkins Co.)

2. Hertz, R (1963). Pituitary independence of the prepubertal development of the ovary of the rat and rabbit and its pertinence of the hypoovarianism in women. In: Grady, HG and Smith, DE (eds.) "The Ovary". p.48. (Baltimore: Williams & Wilkins Co.)
3. Lunenfeld, B and Eshkol, A (1970). Immunology of follicle stimulating hormone and luteinizing hormone. Vitamins & Hormones, 27, 131
4. Gougeon, A (1985). Origin and growth of the preovulatory follicle(s) in spontaneous and stimulated cycles. In: Testart, J and Frydman, R. (eds.) "Human In Vitro Fertilization"; Inserm Symposium No.24, p.3. (Elsevier Science Publisher, B.V.)
5. Baker, TG (1982). Oogenesis and ovulation in germ cells and fertilization. In: Austin, CR and Short, RV (eds.) "Reproduction in Mammals" Vol.1. p.17 (Cambridge University Press)
6. diZerega, GS, Turner, CK, Stouffer, RL, and Hodgen, GD (1981). Suppression of follicle stimulating hormone dependent folliculogenesis during the prime ovarian cycles. J Clin Endocrinol Metab, 52, 451
7. Ross, GT, Cargille, CM, Lipsett, MB, Rayford, PL, Marshall, JR, Strott, CA, and Rodbard, D (1970). Pituitary and gonadal hormones in women during spontaneous and induced ovulatory cycles. Rec Prog Horm Res, 26, 1
8. Landgren, BM, Unden, AL, and Dicsfalusy, E (1980). Hormonal profile of the cycle in 68 normally menstruating women. Acta Endocrinol, 94, 89
9. Lewinthal, D, Furman, A, Blankstein, J and Lunenfeld, B (1986). Stable abnormalities in follicular development and hormonal profile in women with unexplained infertility. Fertil Steril, 46, 833
10. Insler, V and Lunenfeld, B (1974). Application of human gonadotropin for induction of ovulation. In: Campos da Paz, A, Hasegawa, T, Notake, Y and Hayashi, M (eds.) "Human Reproduction". p.25. (Tokyo: Igaku Shoin)
11. Insler, V and Lunenfeld, B (1977). Human gonadotropins. In: Philip, EE, Barnes, J and Newton, M (eds.) "Scientific Foundation of Obstetrics and Gynaecology" p.629. (London: Heinemann)
12. Goodman, AL, Nixon, WE, Johnson, DL and Hodgen, GD (1977). Regulation of folliculogenesis in the rhesus monkey: selection of the dominant follicle. Endocrinology, 100, 155
13. Hodgen GD (1982). The dominant follicle. Fertil Steril, 38, 281
14. Hodgen, GD, Goodman, AL, Stouffer, RL, Williams, RF, di Zerega, GS, Kreitman, OL, Marut, EL and Schenken, RS (1983). Selection of the dominant follicle and its ovum in the menstrual cycle. In: Baier, HM and Lindner, HR (eds.) "Fertilization of the Human Egg In Vitro". p.57. (Springer, Berlin)
15. Blankstein, J, Mashiach, S, and Lunenfeld, B (1986) (eds.). "Ovulation Induction and In Vitro Fertilization". (Year Book Medical Publishers, Inc)

16. Bringer, J, Hedon, B, Gibert, F, et al (1986). Induction de l'ovulation par injections pulsees de gonadoliberine (GnRH). In: Buvat, J and Bringer, J (eds.) "Induction et Stimulation de l'Ovulation". (Paris: Doin Editeurs)
17. Lunenfeld E, Potashnik, G, and Insler, V (1986). Combined GnRH agonist and gonadotropin therapy in patients who failed to respond to previous ovulation inducting therapy. Israel Fertility Society Meeting, Abst, p.15
18. Diamond, MP (1988). Surgical aspects of infertility. In: Sciarra, JJ (ed.) "Gynecology and Obstetrics", 5, p61

9

PHYSIOLOGIC EFFECTS OF A GONADOTROPIN RELEASING HORMONE ANTAGONIST IN NORMAL WOMEN

Janet E. HALL, Todd D. BRODIE, Tom M. BADGER, Jean RIVIER, Wylie VALE, P. Michael CONN and William F. CROWLEY, Jr.
Reproductive Endocrine Unit and the Vincent Memorial Research Laboratories; the Departments of Medicine and Gynecology, Massachusetts General Hospital, Boston, Massachusetts 02114; The Salk Institute for Biological Studies, La Jolla, California 92037; and the Department of Pharmacology, University of Iowa College of Medicine, Iowa City, Iowa 52242, USA

INTRODUCTION

Because of their unique ability to cause pituitary desensitization [1], agonist analogs of GnRH have been used successfully to block gonadotropin output in the therapy of hormone sensitive tumors [2, 3] and other sex-steroid dependent diseases such as endometriosis [4] and uterine leiomyoma [5], as well as in precocious puberty [6]. However, the complexity of action of these agonist analogs limits their use as physiologic probes. Additionally, the initial agonist phase prior to desensitization is not optimal for therapeutic uses in certain settings [2, 3]. Pure antagonists to the action of GnRH have now been developed which block the effect of GnRH on gonadotropin release in pituitary cell cultures [7], perifused pituitary cell columns [8] and intact animals [7, 9, 10]. These GnRH antagonists have been shown to compete with GnRH for receptor binding [11-15], but to stimulate receptor internalization at a slower rate than GnRH or its super-agonist analogs and to be processed differently [8, 16, 17].

We have studied one of the GnRH antagonists, [N-Ac-D-Nal(2)^1,D-pF-Phe^2,D-Trp^3,D-Arg^6]GnRH (the NAL-ARG GnRH antagonist), in normal women in the early follicular phase of the menstrual cycle. This antagonist has been shown to block the action of GnRH effectively in 'in vitro' and 'in vivo' animal studies [7]. We have examined the responses of both LH and FSH to administration of the NAL-ARG GnRH antagonist over a log order of doses.

METHODS

Studies were performed in healthy women in the early follicular phase of the menstrual cycle (day 2 to 5 from the onset of menstruation). Subjects were between the ages of 18 and 40 and all had a history of regular menstrual cycles of 25 to 35 days and had ovulated in the cycle prior to study as assessed by a midluteal phase plasma progesterone level of >6ng/ml and/or a biphasic basal body temperature chart. None of the subjects had a prior history of allergy to drugs and none had used hormonal medications for a minimum of three months prior to study. All subjects had either undergone a prior tubal ligation or consented to the careful use of an effective method of contraception during the month of study and none of the subjects were pregnant at the time of study.

The study was approved by the Subcommittee on Human Studies of the Massachusetts General Hospital and a signed informed consent was obtained from each subject.

All studies were conducted in the Clinical Research Center at the Massachusetts General Hospital. The studies were begun at 8 am and subjects were not allowed to sleep for the first 12 hours due to the known sleep-related slowing of LH pulses characteristic of the early follicular phase [18, 19]. Following verification of a negative beta-HCG, an intravenous catheter was inserted into an antecubital vein for blood sampling and kept patent with heparinized saline. Prior to each study, subjects demonstrated a negative scratch test with 1μg of the NAL-ARG GnRH antagonist and each subject received Benadryl (25mg i.m.) one hour prior to subcutaneous administration of the antagonist. Each study consisted of 4 hours of baseline blood sampling and a further 24 hours of blood sampling following administration of the GnRH antagonist. Blood was sampled every 10 minutes for the first 12 hours (4 hours pre- and 8 hours post-antagonist administration) and hourly for the remainder of the study. The NAL-ARG GnRH antagonist was administered subcutaneously at doses of 50μg/kg (6 subjects), 150μg/kg (6 subjects) and 500μg/kg (5 subjects) A total of 13 women were studied with four subjects studied on two occasions at least two months apart. No subject received a given dose of antagonist on more than one occasion.

LH and FSH were measured in all samples. Estradiol and progesterone were assessed at 4 hourly intervals and routine chemistries (hemoglobin, hematocrit, white blood cell count, platelet count, SGOT, alkaline phosphatase, BUN and creatinine) were measured at the onset and completion of the study. Vital signs were monitored at regular intervals throughout the study and every 15 minutes around the time of antagonist administration.

Plasma samples were measured for estradiol, progesterone, LH and FSH by radioimmunossay as previously described [20]. Serum antagonist levels were determined by radioimmunoassay using an antiserum produced in rabbits using a GnRH antagonist conjugated to keyhole limpet hemocyanin. The cross-reactivity was <0.2% with GnRH and <0.01% with [D-Lys^6]-GnRH, [des-pyroGlu^1]-GnRH or [desGly^{10}]-GnRH, TRH, arginine vasopressin, LH, GH, PRL and somatostatin. The sensitivity of the assay was 0.2ng/tube with an intra-assay coefficient of variation of 1.6 to 9% and an inter-assay coefficient of variation of 12%.

Analysis of pulsatile LH secretion was performed using a modification of the Santen and Bardin method [21] whereby each pulse was required to consist of two points in which the nadir to peak was greater than 20% of baseline and at least one point had an absolute amplitude of 2 mIU/ml. Three four-hour time periods, consisting of the four hour baseline time period and the first and second four hours following antagonist administration, were used for analysis of pulsatile LH secretion. The effect of antagonist administration on LH pulse characteristics was compared to baseline using the exact signed rank test for frequency comparisons and paired t-tests for amplitude comparisons. Comparisons between baseline and post antagonist hormone levels were made using non- paired t-tests or Mann-Whitney U tests where applicable. The percent inhibition in response to antagonist administration was calculated by expressing the difference between the mean of the 6 consecutive points (1 hour) which constituted the nadir following antagonist administration and the mean baseline value, as a percentage of baseline. Apparent plasma disappearance of serum antagonist levels was assessed by assuming a single exponential function and fitting a line to the log of the concentration over time. Analysis of variance and one-way analysis of variance were used to determine differences in the slopes between doses.

Results are expressed as the mean +/- sem and, unless specified, the 0.05 level was construed as the minimum level of significance throughout.

RESULTS

At all doses, peak serum concentrations of the antagonist were present within the first 30 minutes following subcutaneous administration of the NAL-ARG GnRH antagonist, reaching levels of 7.5 +/- 2.1ng/ml, 20.4 +/- 6.1ng/ml and 151.0 +/ 21.1ng/ml at doses of 50, 150 and 500μg/kg, respectively. Serum antagonist levels, as assessed by radioimmunoassay, were well-maintained with the apparent plasma disappearance half-life calculated as 8.8 +/- 1.5 hr. The threshold of serum antagonist concentration for LH suppression was approximately 6ng/ml with resumption of pulses seen at concentrations below this level.

Analysis of LH pulse characteristics over the portion of the study in which blood was sampled at 10 minute intervals demonstrated no significant differences in LH pulse frequency or amplitude between the baseline sampling periods for the three groups. However, dose-dependent changes in the pulsatile characteristics of LH secretion were apparent following administration of the NAL-ARG GnRH antagonist (Fig. 1). With the administration of 50μg/kg, a nonsignificant ($p<0.07$) decrease in pulse frequency was evident in the first four hours with return to baseline in the second four hours, while there was no change in LH pulse amplitude. Following a dose of 150ug/kg, both frequency ($p<0,03$) and amplitude ($p<0.03$) of LH pulses decreased initially with return of frequency to baseline in the second four hours, while pulse amplitude remained suppressed. Administration of a dose of 500μg/kg of the antagonist produced a decrease in LH pulse frequency ($p<0.03$) and amplitude which was sustained for both post antagonist frequent sampling periods.

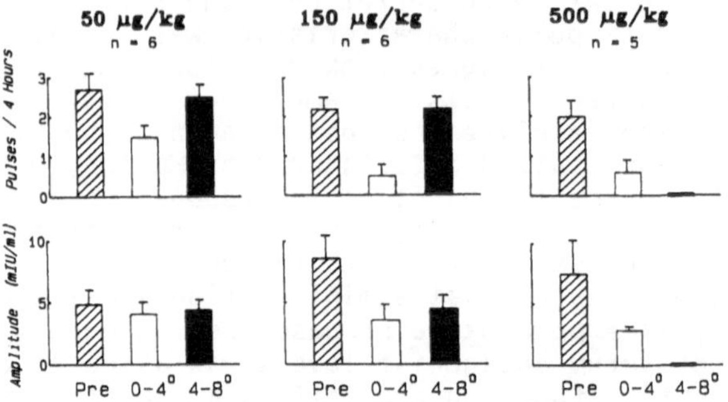

FIGURE 1 Frequency (upper panel) and amplitude (lower panel) of LH pulses assessed in the four hours pre- and the first and second four hours post administration of the GnRH agonist at the doses indicated. See text for description of statistical comparisons

Changes in pulsatile LH secretion were reflected in significant decreases in mean levels of LH at all doses examined ($p<0.001$, Fig. 2). At all doses, the nadir or point of maximum LH suppression had been achieved by three hours following antagonist administration. However, the duration of suppression was markedly influenced by administered dose. Recovery to baseline occurred by 12 hours following administration of 50μg/kg and by 18 hours with administration of 150μg/kg, but full recovery to baseline had not occurred 24 hours following the 500μg/kg dose.

In striking contrast to the changes in LH, FSH was relatively unchanged following administration of the NAL-ARG-GnRH antagonist (Fig. 3). The differential effect of GnRH antagonist administration on LH and FSH is even more apparent when the maximum degree of gonadotropin suppression is expressed as a percent decrease from baseline. For LH, this increased from 40% at 50μg/kg to 60% at 150μg/kg, but there was no further increase at the 500μg/kg dose (Fig. 4). Due to the longer half life of FSH, the maximum suppressive effect of the GnRH antagonist would not be expected to be apparent until at least 8 hours

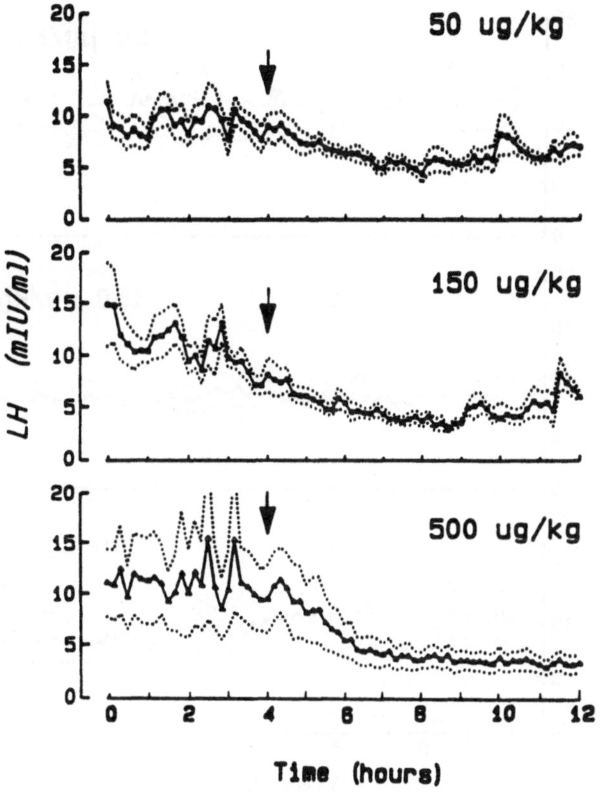

FIGURE 2 Mean (solid line) +/- 1 sem (dotted lines) for serum LH over the first 12 hr of the study at the doses indicated. The arrow indicates the timing of antagonist administration

following administration. Comparison of values obtained in the 7-8 hour time period following antagonist administration with baseline revealed suppression of 15 +/- 9%, 4 +/- 4% and 16 +/- 5% for doses of 50, 150 and 500μg/kg, respectively. No greater changes were seen at any timepoint over the full 24 hr following antagonist administration.

Baseline levels of estradiol and progesterone were 32.2 +/- 4.1pg/ml and 1.11 +/- 0.35ng/ml, respectively, within the normal range for subjects in the early follicular phase of the menstrual cycle [18]. There was no significant difference in baseline levels between subjects tested at the three different doses and no consistent changes in either ovarian steroid hormone, measured at

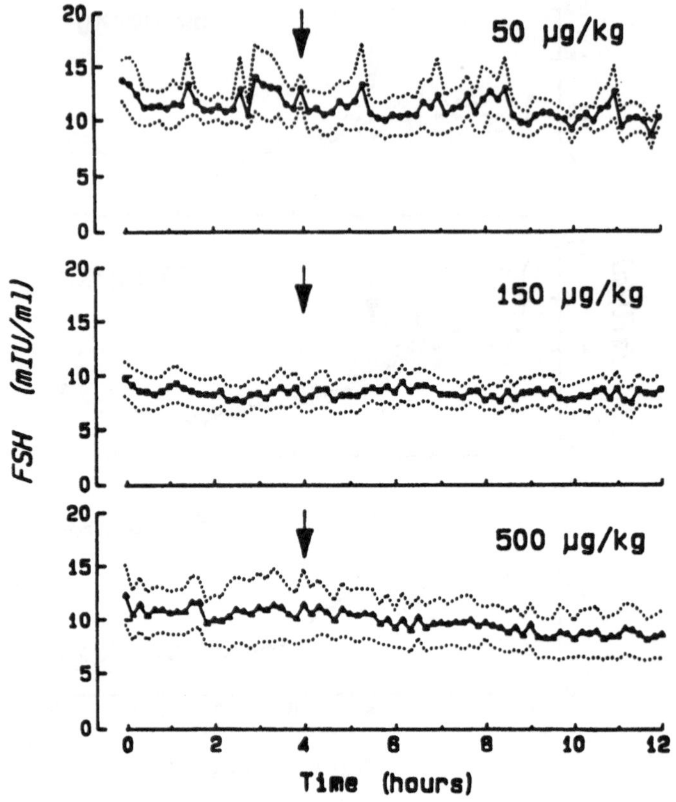

FIGURE 3 Mean (solid line) +/- 1 sem (dotted lines) for serum FSH overthe first 12 hr of the study at the doses indicated. The arrow indicates the timing of antagonist administration

4 hr intervals, in response to antagonist administration at any of the three doses tested.

There was no significant change in hemoglobin, white blood cell count or platelet count from the beginning to the completion of the study at any of the antagonist doses tested. Indices of hepatic and renal function remained unchanged and there was no change in vital signs in response to antagonist administration. Each subject experienced local induration, erythema and tenderness at the site of subcutaneous injection of the antagonist. Which was not dose dependent, in spite of prior antihistamine administration. Three subjects developed urticarial reactions which were distinct from the local reactions. The urticarial reactions were confined to the anterior chest or abdomen, began

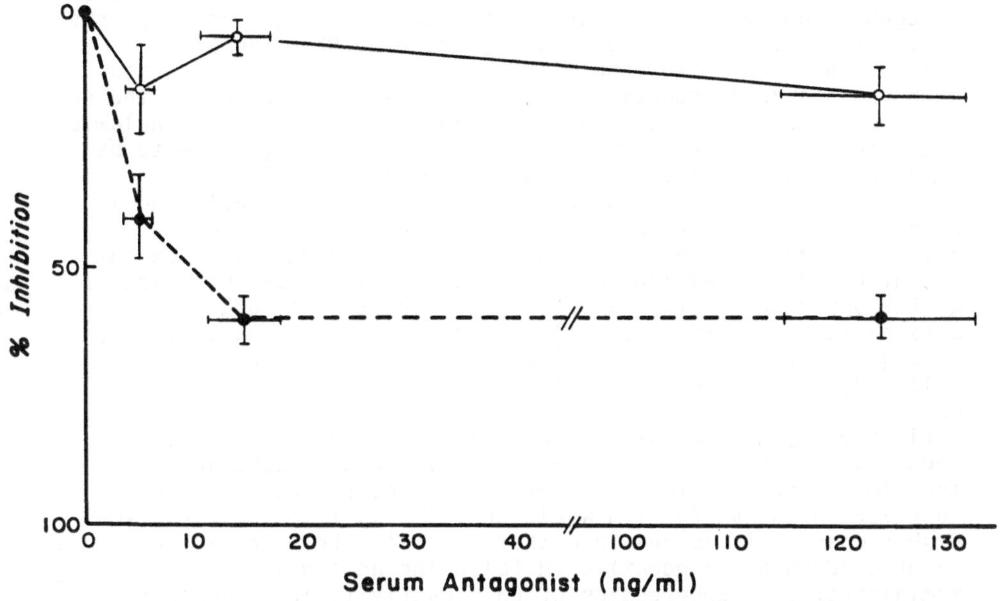

FIGURE 4 Mean +/- sem of the percent inhibition of LH (o--o) and FSH (o--o) in relation to serum antagonist levels (mean +/- sem on the horizontal axis for doses of 50, 150 and 500µ/kg)

within 15 minutes of antagonist administration and resolved spontaneously within 90 minutes with no further therapy. There were no associated changes in vital signs and no symptoms suggestive of respiratory compromise. All such reactions were experienced in association with administration of the 500µg/kg dose of the NAL-ARG GnRH antagonist. Analysis of the three individual cases suggests that both administered dose and a prior history of urticarial reactions to other stimulants may have been etiologic factors.

DISCUSSION

The present studies demonstrate that a single subcutaneous injection of the NAL-ARG GnRH antagonist immediately and effectively suppresses LH levels in women studied in the early follicular phase of the menstrual cycle. In this model, the analysis of pulsatile secretion of LH provides a direct parameter of blockade of the effect of endogenous GnRH. Both the amplitude and frequency of LH pulses was decreased in a dose-dependent manner following institution of GnRH blockade. The observation of a decrease in LH pulse frequency at lower doses of this pure pituitary GnRH-receptor blocker may suggest that endogenous pulses of GnRH of decreased quantity may not be transmitted as LH pulses in the face of mild to moderate degrees of GnRH antagonism. Evidence of such subthreshold or 'blocked' pulses of endogenous GnRH was initially suggested by portal sampling studies in the ewe in which it was demonstrated that some pulses of the hypothalamic releasing factor appeared to be of insufficient magnitude to be translated as LH pulses by the anterior pituitary [22].

Alterations in LH pulse characteristics were reflected in mean LH levels and the duration of LH suppression following antagonist administration was also dose dependent. The maximum amount of LH suppression that could be achieved was 60% which is at the upper end of the range of LH suppression by GnRH antagonists reported previously in animal and human studies [9, 23-25]. This failure of total suppression of LH secretion following GnRH antagonist administration is puzzling. The observation that the maximal degree of suppression of LH was not influenced by an increase in GnRH antagonist dose from 150 to 500μg/kg, which was accompanied by a marked and sustained increase in serum antagonist levels, suggests that a further increase in LH suppression would be unlikely to occur with even higher doses. It is possible that bioactive LH is relatively more suppressed than immunoactive LH following antagonist administration. Suppression of LH bioactivity in response to other GnRH antagonists has been found to occur to a greater degree than immunoactivity in one study in men [24], but this was not confirmed in a study in postmenopausal women [26]. It is also possible that the remaining LH measured in the serum by radioimmunoassay results from cross-reactivity of remaining free alpha subunit with the LH antibody. Although the cross-reactivity of the LH antibody with the alpha subunit in the assays reported herein is < 4% [20], this cross-reactivity may assume a more significant role in the total absence of endogenous LH secretion. In contrast to the significant suppression produced by GnRH antagonist administration, there was a relatively small degree of suppression of plasma FSH levels in women in the early follicular phase of the menstrual cycle. These findings are in agreement with previous reports of FSH responses to acute GnRH antagonist administration in animals [9, 27, 28] and in man [23-26] as well as with the differential response of LH and FSH observed in rats following administration of GnRH antisera [29]. It is possible that a longer duration of frequent blood sampling may have unmasked a greater degree of suppression of FSH due to its longer half-life relative to LH [30, 31]. However, more significant changes should have been observable in the hourly sampling portion of the study if this hypothesis were true. In addition, a longer duration of GnRH blockade might produce a greater effect on FSH secretion if the primary GnRH effect on FSH is on hormone synthesis rather than merely on release of hormone from intracellular stores. Alternatively, the differential gonadotropin response to GnRH antagonism may reflect a different threshold of the anterior pituitary for GnRH induction of FSH release. As with LH, it is also possible that bioactive FSH is suppressed to a greater degree than is immunoactive FSH [32]. Finally, this differential effect of GnRH antagonism on the two gonadotropins may well point to a separate releasing factor responsible for at least some control of FSH secretion as suggested by the recent discovery of an ovarian FSH releasing peptide [33, 34].

In our studies, levels of ovarian hormones were unaffected by the transient blockade of gonadotropins unlike the effects on testosterone seen in similar studies in men [24]. In the early follicular phase of the menstrual cycle, follicular development and the production of estradiol are largely controlled by FSH which was relatively unaffected over the duration of GnRH blockade in the present study. Therefore, the lack of change in sex steroids may not be surprising.

Serum antagonist levels as assessed by radioimmunoassay remained elevated for a significant period of time. It is possible that this lack of rapid degradation reflects not only the structural modifications which protect these compounds from rapid proteolysis and thus prolong their acton at the GnRH receptor, but also significant binding to plasma proteins. This latter explanation has been previously proposed for potent GnRH antagonists [26]. However, it is also possible that the prolonged apparent serum disappearance represents a degree of cross-reactivity with metabolites of the GnRH antagonist as has recently been demonstrated for growth hormone releasing factor [35].

Many of the antagonists to GnRH which have now been synthesized produce histamine release in 'in vitro' studies [36], and other histamine-mediated side effects have been observed in animals administered high concentrations of certain antagonists [37]. Because of these effects in pre-clinical trials, a scratch test was administered to all subjects prior to antagonist administration and an antihistamine was used prior to each study. Despite these precautions, urticarial reactions were experienced by three of the subjects tested which are almost certain to have been histamine mediated. All the urticarial reactions occurred at the highest doses and the range of serum levels between the doses which effectively block GnRH and those which are associated with the development of urticaria did not overlap. While it may be that the therapeutic index will permit the safe use of the NAL-ARG GnRH antagonist in carefully selected circumstances, developmental work is continuing in several laboratories in an effort to reduce histamine-related side-effects in future generations of GnRH antagonists.

This study demonstrates that subcutaneous administration of a GnRH antagonist rapidly and effectively antagonizes the action of GnRH in a dose-dependent manner. A single injection of this antagonist produces a differential suppression of LH and FSH adding support to the concept of at least some independence of FSH from GnRH control and suggesting that the antagonist treated female may serve as a model for the investigation of GnRH-independent control of FSH.

ACKNOWLEDGEMENTS

We would like to thank Dr. Michael Blank and Hazelton Laboratories for performing the serum antagonist assays and the nurses of the Clinical Research Center for their help with the clinical studies.

REFERENCES

1. Bhasin, S, and Swerdloff, RS (1986). Mechanisms of gonadotropin-releasing hormone agonist action in the human male. Endocr Rev, 7, 106

2. Labrie, F, Dupont, A, Belanger, A, St-Arnaud, R, Giguere, M, Lacourciere, Y, Emond, J and Monfette, G (1986). Treatment of prostate cancer with gonadotropin-releasing hormone agonists. Endocr Rev, 7, 67

3. Manni, A, Santen, R, Harvey, H, Lipton, A and Max, D (1986). Treatment of breast cancer with gonadotropin-releasing hormone. Endocr Rev, 7, 89

4. Schriock,E, Monroe, SE, Henzl, M and Jaffe, RJ (1985). Treatment of endometriosis with a potent agonist of gonadotropin-releasing hormone (nafarelin). Fertil Steril, 44, 583

5. Healey, DL, Lawson, SR, Abbott, M, Baird, DT and Fraser, HM (1986). Toward removing uterine fibroids without surgery: subcutaneous infusion of a luteinizing hormone-releasing hormone agonist commencing in the luteal phase. J Clin Endocrinol Metab, 63, 619

6. Boepple, PA, Mansfield, MJ, Wierman, ME, Rudlin, CR, Bode, HH, Crigler, JF Jr, Crawford, JD and Crowley, WF Jr (1986). Use of a potent, long acting agonist of gonadotropin-releasing hormone in the treatment of precocious puberty. Endocr Rev, 7, 24

7. Rivier, C, Rivier, J, Perrin, M and Vale, W (1983). Comparison of the effect of several gonadotropin releasing hormone antagonists on luteinizing hormone secretion, receptor binding and ovulation. Biol Reprod, 29, 374

8. Smith, WA and Conn, PM (1983). GnRH-mediated desensitization of the pituitary gonadotrope is not calcium dependent. Endocrinology, 112, 408

9. Grady, RR, Shin, L, Charlesworth, MC, Cohen-Becker, IR, Smith, M, Rivier, C, Rivier, J, Vale, W and Schwartz, N (1985). Differential suppression of follicle-stimulating hormone secretion in vivo by a gonadotropin-releasing hormone antagonist. Neuroendocrinology, 40, 246

10. Pineda, JL, Lee, BC, Spiliotis, BE, Vale, W, Rivier, J, Brown, TJ and Bercu, BB (1980). Effect of GnRH antagonist, $(Ac\Delta^{3}Pro^{1},pFDPhe^{2},DTrp^{3,6})$GnRH, on pulsatile gonadotropin secretion in the castrate male primate. J Clin Endocrinol Metab, 56, 420

11. Clayton, RN and, Catt, KJ (1980). Receptor-binding affinity of gonadotropin-releasing hormone analogs: analysis of radiologand-receptor assay. J Clin Endocrinol Metab, 106, 1154

12. Loumay, E, Wynn, PC, Coy, D and Catt, KJ (1984). Receptor-binding properties of gonadotropin-releasing hormone derivatives. J Biol Chem, 259, 12663
13. Marian, J, Cooper, RL and Conn, PM (1981). Regulation of the rat pituitary gonadotropin-releasing hormone receptor. Mol Pharmacol, 19, 399
14. Perrin, MH, Haas, Y, Rivier, J and Vale, WW (1983). Gonadotropin-releasing hormone binding to rat anterior pituitary membrane homogenates: comparison of antagonists and agonists using radiolabeled antagonist and agonist. Mol Pharmacol, 23, 44
15. Perrin, MH, Rivier, J and Vale, WW (1980). Radioligand assay for gonadotropin-releasing hormone: relative potencies of agonists and antagonists. Endocrinology, 106, 1289
16. Jennes, L, Coy, D and Conn, PM (1986). Receptor-mediated uptake of GnRH agonist and antagonists by cultured gonadotropes: evidence for differential intracellular routing. Peptides, 7, 459
17. Wynn, PC, Suarez-Quian, CA, Childs, GV and Catt, KJ (1986). Pituitary binding and internalization of radioiodinated gonadotropin-releasing hormone agonist and antagonist ligands in vitro and in vivo. Endocrinology, 111, 1852
18. Filicori, M, Santoro, N, Merriam, GR and Crowley, WF (1986). Characterization of the physiological pattern of episodic gonadotropin secretion throughout the human menstrual cycle. J Clin Endocrinol Metab, 62, 1136
19. Soules, MR, Steiner, RA, Cohen, NL, Bremner, WJ and Clifton, DK (1985). Nocturnal slowing of pulsatile luteinizing hormone secretion in women during the follicular phase of the menstrual cycle. J Clin Endocrinol Metab, 61, 43
20. Filicori, M, Butler, JP and Crowley, WF (1984). Neuroendocrine regulation of the corpus luteum in the human. J Clin Invest, 73, 1638
21. Santen, RJ and Bardin, CW (1973). Episodic luteinizing hormone secretion in man. Pulse analysis, clinical interpretation, physiologic mechanisms. J Clin Invest, 52, 2617
22. Clarke, IJ and Cummins, JT (1982). The temporal relationship between gonadotropin releasing hormone (GnRH) and luteinizing hormone (LH) secretion in ovariectomized ewes. Endocrinology, 111, 1737
23. Cetel, NS, Rivier, J, Vale, W and Yen, SSC (1983). The dynamics of gonadotropin inhibition of women induced by an antagonistic analog of gonadotropin-releasing hormone. J Clin Endocrinol Metab, 57, 62
24. Mais, V, Kazer, RR, Cetel, NS, Rivier, J, Vale, W and Yen, SSC (1986). The dependency of folliculogenesis and corpus luteum function on pulsatile gonadotropin secretion in cycling women using a gonadotropin-releasing hormone antagonist as a probe. J Clin Endocrinol Metab, 62, 1250
25. Pavlou, SN, Debold, CR, Island, DP, Wakefield, G, Rivier, J, Vale, W, and Rabin D (1986). Single subcutaneous doses of a luteinizing hormone-releasing hormone antagonist suppress serum gonadotropin and testosterone levels in normal men. J Clin Endocrinol Metab, 63, 303

26. Davis, M, Veldhuis, JD, Rogol, AD, Dufau, ML and Catt, KJ (1987). Sustained inhibitory actions of a potent antagonist of gonadotropin-releasing hormone (GnRH) in post-menopausal women. J Clin Endocrinol Metab, 64, 1268
27. de Paolo, LV (1985). Differential regulation of pulsatile luteinizing hormone (LH) and follicle-stimulating hormone secretion in ovariectomized rats disclosed by treatment with a LH-releasing hormone antagonist and phenobarbital. J Clin Endocrinol Metab, 117, 1826
28. Heber, D, Dodson, R and Swerdloff, RS (1982). Pituitary receptor site blockade by a gonadotropin-releasing hormone antagonist in vivo: mechanism of action. Science, 216, 420
29. Culler, MD and Negro-Vilar, A (1986). Evidence that pulsatile follicle-stimulating hormone secretion is independent of endogenous luteinizing hormone-releasing hormone. J Clin Endocrinol Metab, 118, 609
30. Coble, YD, Kohler, PO, Cargille, CM and Ross, GT (1969). Production rates and metabolic clearance rates of human follicle-stimulating hormone in premenopausal and postmenopausal women. J Clin Invest, 48, 359
31. Yen, SSC, Llerena, LA, Pearson, OH and Littell, AS (1970). Disappearance rates of endogenous follicle-stimulating hormone in serum following surgical hypophysectomy in man. J Clin Endocrinol Metab, 30, 325
32. Dahl, KD, Pavlou, SN, Kovacs, WJ and Hsueh, AJW (1986). The changing ratio of serum bioactive to immunoreactive follicle-stimulating hormone in normal men following treatment with a potent gonadotropin releasing hormone antagonist. J Clin Endocrinol Metab, 63, 792
33. Vale, W, Rivier, J, Vaughan, J, McClintock, R, Corrigan, A, Woo, W, Karr, D and Spiess, J (1986). Purification and characterization of an FSH releasing protein from porcine ovarian follicular fluid. Nature, 321, 776
34. Ling, N, Ying, S-Y, Ueno, N, Shimasaki, S, Esch, F, Hotta, M and Guillemin, R (1986). Pituitary FSH is released by a heterodimer of the beta-subunits from the two forms of inhibin. Nature, 321, 779
35. Frohman, LA, Downs, TR, Williams, TC, Heimer, EP, Pan, Y-CE and Felix, AM (1986). Rapid enzymatic degradation of growth hormone-releasing hormone by plasma in vitro and in vivo to a biologically inactive product cleaved at the NH_2 terminus. J Clin Invest, 78, 906
36. Hook, WA, Karten, M and Siraganian, RP (1985). Histamine release by structural analogs of LHRH. Fed Proc, 44, 1323
37. Schmidt, F, Sundaram, K, Thau, RB and Bardin, CW (1984). (Ac-D-$NAL2^1$,4FD-Phe^2,D-Trp^3,D-Arg^6)-LHRH, a potent antagonist of LHRH, produces transient edema and behavioral changes in rats. Contraception, 29, 283

10
PHARMACOLOGICAL HYPOGONADOTROPISM CAN BE USED TO ADVANTAGE FOR OVULATION INDUCTION PROTOCOLS

G. BETTENDORF, W. BRAENDLE, Ch. LINDNER, V. LICHTENBERG, M. LUCKHARDT and T. SCHLOTFELD
Abteilung fuer klinische und experimentelle Endokrinologie
der Universitaets-Frauenklinik, Martinistrasse 52, 2000 Hamburg 20, FRG

INTRODUCTION

Ovarian stimulation with hMG/hCG is an established therapeutic principle in anovulatory patients with amenorrhea, low gonadotropins and a negligible endogenous estrogen production. Exogenous gonadotropins are also used for ovarian stimulation in women who are not typical candidates for this type of treatment, i.e. those with anovulatory cycles and in cases of luteal insufficiency which do not respond to clomiphene. In addition, exogenous gonadotropins are given to patients who are to be prepared for intrauterine insemination, in vitro fertilization (IVF) or gamete intrafallopian transfer (GIFT) in order to achieve multifollicular development.

As early as the 1960s, when the first patients were treated with gonadotropins, it became evident that women with hypogonadotropism were the ideal candidates for this treatment design, i.e. they had the highest pregnancy rates. The more severe the lack of endogenous gonadotropins the better was the patient's chance to conceive during therapy with human Menopausal Gonadotropins (hMG).

The reason for the poor results in cyclic insufficiency is the irregular and unpredictable hypothalamo-pituitary response during exogenous stimulation. The increased amounts of estrogens produced by the hyperstimulated ovaries do not reduce the ability of the pituitary to respond to their positive feed back-action. It has been shown that in many stimulation cycles irregular fluctuations occur in LH as well as early luteinization and premature LHsurges. In clinical practice this means that careful monitoring by E2 measurement and ultrasonography does not provide a complete picture of the endocrine situation. This complicates the exact timing of injection of hCG to induce ovulation. In addition, a consequence of the increasing estrogen levels the pituitary may react with a release of LH at a time before complete follicular maturation is achieved, resulting in premature luteinization. In these cycles the probability of fertilization is low. The phenomenon of surges of endogenous LH was initially noticed when human pituitary gonadotropin alone was used for induction of ovulation [1]. Later, careful endocrine monitoring of hMG stimulation cycles, especially in patients prepared for IVF [2], showed unpredictable rises of progesterone and LH prior to the injection of hCG, providing explanations for the poor success rate.

FIRST EXPERIENCES

Early experiments had shown that ovarian stimulation with exogenous gonadotropins was possible in patients concomitantly treated with an estrogen/progesterone combination [3]. We hypothesised that this induced a time-limited blockade of pituitary function, resulting in a resting ovarian function which gave better conditions for exogenous stimulation. However, ovarian steroids should not be used for this purpose because of their effects on the endometrium. Therefore, we used Danazol to mimic the hypogonadotropic state. In this situation ovarian stimulation by hMG was evoked and ovulation could be induced, but it was also noticed that the cervical glands were suppressed, even in the presence of high endogenous estrogen activity [4].

Later experiments used the GnRH analogue (GnRH-A) buserelin (Hoechst AG, Frankfurt A.M., FRG) to induce a selective pituitary desensitization [5]. Buserelin caused initial stimulation of gonadotropins then FSH and later LH levels were suppressed. When hMG was administered ovarian stimulation could be induced. At that time hMG and Buserelin treatments were started simultaneously. The clinical results were disappointing and the pregnancy rate was low. It was suggested that the degree of pituitary suppression was not complete. Therefore, we changed our protocol. Starting in the early follicular phase, buserelin was administered intranasally four times per day for a total dose of 1.2 mg per day. FSH, LH and estrogen levels were measured periodically, and pituitary responsiveness was tested. This was done by two procedures: first by measuring endogenous fluctuation in LH and second by performing an LH-provocation test with estradiol involving 1 mg E2-benzoate injected intramusculary and measurement of the LH reaction 48 hours later (E2-test). Negative LH fluctuation was defined as LH variation below two standard deviations of intraassay variation and negative E-2-test as no similarly defined LH increase 48 hours after E2-benzoate injection. Ovarian stimulation was initiated only when both tests were negative indicating complete pituitary unresponsiveness. Buserelin-treatment was continued during ovarian stimulation and after ovulation during the luteal phase until a positive pregnancy-test was noted or menstrual bleeding occurred.

In a first study we treated 12 women with buserelin before ovarian stimulation for IVF was started [6]. In all of these patients a previous IVF stimulation cycle had been cancelled because of an endogenous LH surge and premature luteinization hMG stimulation for IVF was again started as soon as complete pituitary suppression was achieved. As shown in Table 1 no spontaneous LH surges occurred. There was an increased amount of

Table 1. HMG stimulation for IVF without and with LHRH-A pretreatment in the same patients.

	hMG/hCG	Buserelin/hMG/hCG	P
Patients	12	12	
Cycles	12	12	
Premature LH-surge	12	0	<0.001
LH(IU/l)[a]	22.5 ± 16.6	4.5 ± 1.1	<0.01
P (ng/ml)[a]	1.9 ± 1.6	0.5 ± 0.3	<0.05
E (μg/24 hrs urine)[a]	226 ± 190	242 ± 180	NS
HMG (ampouls)[b]	23.4 ± 5.7	28.9 ± 7.4	<0.05
Ovum pickup	0	12	<0.001
Pregnancies	-	4	

[a]LH, progesterone and estrogen values on the day of hCG application (mean ± SEM).
[b]Amount of hMG used for ovarian stimulation.

hMG required for ovarian stimulation under buserelin treatment. Mean LH and P values on the day of hCG injection were significantly lower, but no difference existed in the urinary estrogens among the stimulation protocols. It was possible to perform successful follicular puncture in all buserelin/hMG cycles and 4 pregnancies resulted. As a consequence we started a second study comparing buserelin/hMG/IVF cycles (43 patients) and conventional hMG/IVF cycles (42 patients). Table 2 summarizes the results in the two groups. Out of 109 started hMG stimulation cycles only 66 follicular punctures could be performed. In 38% premature luteinization occurred: in 2 cases the cause of cancellation was insufficient follicular development. In contrast, oocyte re- trieval was performed in all 74 buserelin/hMG cycles because there was no evidence for a spontaneous LH-surge. The oocyte recovery rate per cycle increased significantly when buserelin was used, as compared with cycles induced with hMG alone. In the combination buserelin/hMG the mean number of oocytes was 5.3 per retrieval, in the hMG cycles 3.8 per retrieval. Moreover the number of oocytes that actually were fertilized was 72% as compared with 52% in the hMG only group. In 97% of the cycles an embryo transfer could be performed with the combined therapy compared to 50% with the conventional therapy. Finally the rate of clinical pregnancies in the buserelin/hMG group was 24% of all treated cycles or 25% of all performed transfers, in the control group 6% per cycle or 11% per embryo transfer (Table 2).

Table 2. IVF results after hMG stimulation without and with LHRH-A pretreatment.

	hMG/hCG		Buserelin/ hMG/hCG		P
	No.	%	No.	%	
Patients	42		43		
Cycles	109	100	74	100	
Premature LH-surge	41/109	38	0/ 74	0	<0.001
Ovum pickup (OPU)	66/109[a]	61	74/ 74	100	<0.001
Oocytes/OPU	251/ 66 (= 3.8)		392/ 74 (= 5.3)		<0.05
Oocytes fertilized	131/251	52	282/392	72	<0.001
Embryo transfer (ET)	54/109	50	72/ 74	97	<0.001
Pregnancies	6/109	6	18/ 74	24	<0.001
Pregnancies/ET	6/ 54	11	18/ 72	25	<0.05

[a]2 cycles were cancelled because of insufficient estrogen rise.

CURRENT DATA

As a consequence of these improved results we have used the same protocol for all ovarian stimulations with hMG/hCG: 1. Induction of ovulation for IVF in patients with clomiphene failure. 2. Ovarian stimulation to prepare patients for intrauterine insemination. 3. Preparing of patients for IVF. 4. Preparing of patients for GIFT.

Induction of pharmacologic hypogonadotropism

In order to improve the pretreatment for pharmacological hypogonadotropism we compared 5 different protocols of LHRH-A application.

Group I (84 patients): buserelin was administered in a total dose of 1.2 mg/day by nasal spray without any other medication. The treatment was started in the early follicular phase of a spontaneous menstrual cycle (day 1-3).

Group II (12 patients): buserelin administration (1.2 mg/day) intranasally) again started in the early follicular phase together with sequential oral contraceptives.

Group III (14 patients): buserelin administration (1.2 mg/day, intranasally) also started in the early follicular phase together with combined oral contraceptives.

Group IV (41 patients): buserelin administration (1.2 mg/day, intranasally) was started in the early luteal phase of a spontaneous menstrual cycle supported by the additional medication of 10 mg Medroxyprogesterone acetate (MPA) for 10 days

Group V (42 patients): In this group we used the LHRH-A Decapeptyl CR (Ferring, Kiel, FRG) as a depot preparation in a single dose of 3.2 mg injected intramuscularly in the early luteal phase of a sponteneous menstrual cycle again supported by 10 mg MPA for 10 days.

Table 3 shows the results of the mean treatment time until complete pituitary desensitization was achieved, proven by a negative E2-test. There was a significant reduction of pretreatment time achieved by the additional medication of a progestin preparation, which was further improved when the LHRH-A application was started in the luteal phase. In all groups we noticed a remarkable individual difference. In addition, the parallel medication of estrogen/progestin combination reduces side effects of estrogen deficiency in hypogonadotropism.

Table 3. Duration of LHRH-A therapy until sufficient pituitary suppression correlated to different treatment protocols.

Group	Mean Time of Treatment Until Proven Gonadotropic Desensitization (Days $\bar{x} \pm$ SEM)	Individual Range (Days)
Group I (n = 84)	41,1 ± 11,7	(15-65)
Group II (n = 12)	27,3 ± 5,5	(14-40)
Group III (n = 14)	25,6 ± 2,1	(13-42)
Group IV (n = 41)	20,7 ± 10,5	(10-51)
Group V (n = 42)	15,1 ± 3,0	(9-25)

Endocrine profiles during LHRH-A treatment

We examined different endocrine parameters during GnRH-A pretreatment before hMG-stimulation. A positive response of LH was found at the beginning of LHRH-A administration. This was most pronounced in groups IV and V in which the treatment was started in the luteal phase. A significant suppression of LH in groups IV and V was found at day 20. In group I this effect was less distinct and the absolute levels of LH remained higher (Fig. 1). In contrast to LH, the FSH levels decreased from the beginning of GnRH-A treatment, reaching the lowest levels at about day 20 in all three groups. The pattern of the LH/FSH ratio

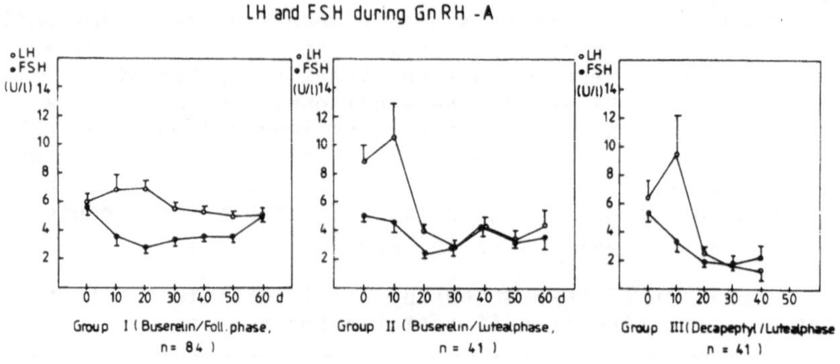

FIGURE 1 Serum gonadotropin values during LHRH-A treatment

demonstrated the differential reaction of the gonadotropins (Fig. 2). Levels of estradiol before GnRH-analogues administration reflect the time of the cycle. During the GnRH-A-medication an increase of E2 was followed by a sharp decrease in all three groups, particularly in groups IV and V. E2 fluctuated around 20 pg/ml or lower. In group I this decrease occurred somewhat later (about day 30-40, Fig. 3A).

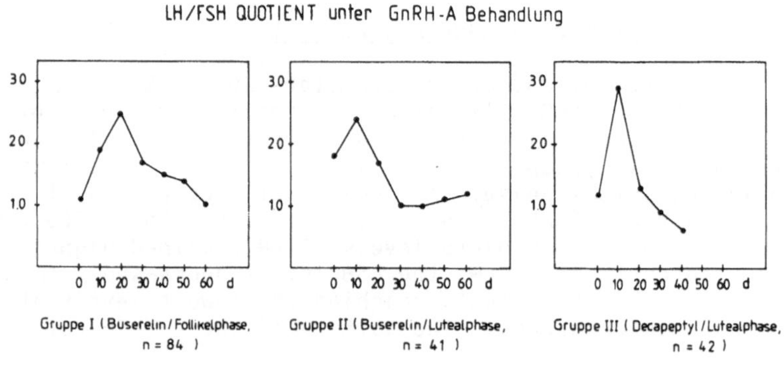

FIGURE 2 LH/FSH ratio during LHRH-A treatment

An interesting finding is the response of the gonadotropins during the E2-test at the time of complete pituitary desensitization. There was no increase of LH following E2 injection, but a decrease which was most pronounced in Group V. FSH showed similar dynamic pattern like LH; again the greatest difference became evident in group V. The relative suppression of FSH was greater than that of LH. Fig. 3B demonstrates a typical profile of gonado- tropin reaction following E2 administration at different times during GnRH-A treatment reflecting the different states of pitui- tary suppression.

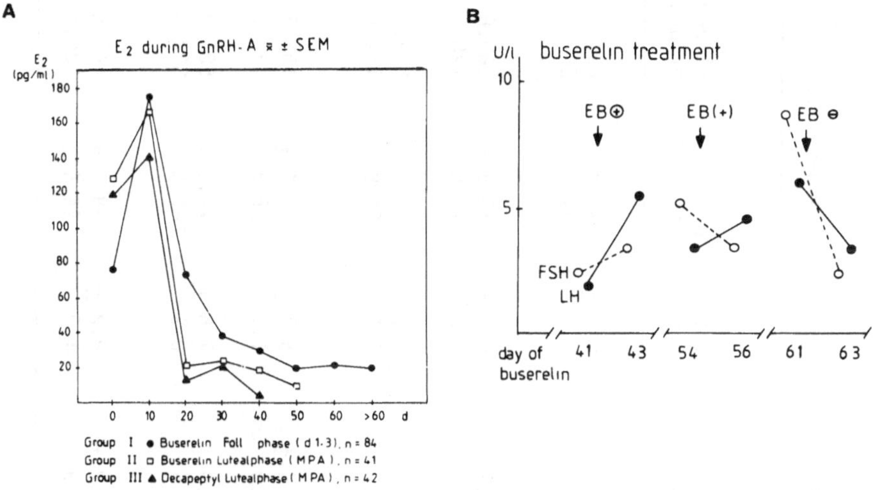

FIGURE 3.A Estradiol levels during LHRH-A treatment.
B. Typical individual profile of estradiol benzoate test during LHRH-A treatment

Ovarian stimulation during pharmacologic hypogonadotropism

The ovarian stimulation period was analyzed according to the two analogues used for pituitary suppression: buserelin and Decapeptyl.

Symptoms of estrogen deficiency were the only side effects noted. Ovarian stimulation was initiated only after pituitary tests were negative, indicating sufficient suppression. The dose of hMG was dependent on the individual response, which was monitored by daily measurement of total estrogens in 24 hour urine collections and by ovarian ultrasonography. Ovulation was induced with hCG 10.000 i.m. when follicles were 18 to 20 mm of diameter and adequate estrogen levels were measured [7].

In each of these groups the cycles were divided into those in which conception occurred and those in which no pregnancy could be achieved. All patients had an infertility of long duration. All of them had cyclic ovarian insufficiency of different degrees

Table 4. Analytical data of hMG, buserelin/hMG and decapeptyl/hMG-cycles.

Treatment	E at Start of hMG	Amp. P. Cycle	Latent Ph. Days	Active Ph. Days	E Increase p. Day in Active Ph.	E at Day of hCG	No. of Foll. >16 at Day of hCG	E/foll.
hMG - hCG pregnant n = 12	13.0 ± 5.9	23.4 ± 8.3	4.8 ± 2.7	5.7 ± 1.7	41.3 ± 37.4	297.1 ± 262	2.2 ± 1.5	76.8 ± 67.9
not pregnant n = 106	13.4 ± 6.8	22.4 ± 5.8	4.1 ± 1.9	6.1 ± 1.8	18.9 ± 14.0	180.8 ± 120	3.5 ± 2.2	51.7 ± 34.3
Buserelin-hMG pregnant n = 17	11.3 ± 2.5	25.4 ± 6.8	4.5 ± 1.8	6.2 ± 0.5	79.7 ± 26.9	522.4 ± 154.8	4.9 ± 3.6	106.6 ± 43
not pregnant n = 75	8.4 ± 2	28.6 ± 9.1	6.4 ± 2.9	5.7 ± 1.1	27.9 ± 26.3	185.7 ± 90.8	3.9 ± 2.8	47.6 ± 32.4
Decapeptyl-hMG pregnant n = 9	9.2 ± 2.6	34.8 ± 8.0	4.9 ± 1.5	7.6 ± 0.9	74.0 ± 46.6	583.2 ± 339.6	7.9 ± 5.5	91.6 ± 75.2
not pregnant n = 33	9.6 ± 6.8	50.9 ± 13.9	7.2 ± 3.3	8.2 ± 1.9	48.6 ± 44.4	445.8 ± 39.8	5.5 ± 3.2	78.5 ± 45.0

or normal ovulatory cycles (prepared for IVF). Those who were hyper- androgenemic before treatment showed normal testosterone levels following LHRH-A. A pathological male factor was found in nearly 40% of the couples and must be borne in mind when reviewing pregnancy rates.

The data of the LHRH-A pretreated patients were compared to the group of patients who were stimulated with hMG/hCG without any pretreatment (Table 4). Basal levels of estrogens were low following LHRH-A pretreatment. The amount of hMG necessary for appropriate ovarian stimulation was dependent on the type of ovarian insufficiency. In earlier studies we reported that the requirement in normogonadotropic amenorrhea was a mean total dose of hMG of 35 ampoules, in hypogonadotropic amenorrhea 47 ampoules, and in cyclic ovarian insufficiency between 20 and 24 ampoules [8]. In this study the same amount as in cyclic ovarian insufficiency was found in the hMG/hCG group, somewhat more in the Buserelin-group, and in the Decapeptyl group 34.8 in conception cycles and 50 in non-conception cycles.

The length of the latent and active phase is a good clinical parameter for the effectiveness of stimulation and ovarian responsiveness. On the basis of all treatment cycles, the latent phase was shortest in the hMG/hCG group but it was similar (four to five days) when only the conception cycles were compared, equal between four and five days.

The active phase was similar in hMG and in Buserelin/hMG treated patients but prolonged in the Decapeptyl-group. As in spontaneous, ovulatory cycles the active phase of follicle development after exogenous ovarian stimulation lasts four to five days. In the combined therapy regimen it is an advantage to extend this time of active follicular growth to allow follicles and oocytes of less maturity to continue their development. LHRH-A combined with hMG allows a greater flexibility of hCG timing since the endogenous gonadotropin activity does not interfere with the exogenous gonadotropin treatment.

The daily increase of estrogens in the active phase was determined. In all three groups this value was less in the nonconception cycles compared to the conception cycles. In the analogue-pretreated patients it was 79 and 74 µg/24 hrs, respectively, in the hMG only group 41 µg/24 hrs, i.e. a steeper slope of the estrogen increase was found in analogue pretreated patients. Moreover, higher levels of estrogens were observed in GnRH-A pretreated patients at the day of hCG injection.

In the hMG/hCG group the mean number of preovulatory follicles at the time of hCG injection as 2.2 and 3.5 in conception versus non-conception cycles, in the buserelin-group 4.9 versus 3.9, in the Decapaptyl-group 7.9 versus 5.5. The larger number of follicles partially explains the higher estrogen level. But it is interesting to see that the estrogen production per follicle in conception cycles is greater than in non-conception cycles and in the analogue pretreated patients greater than during ovarian stimulation with hMG alone. The wide range of the estrogen values demonstrates that there may exist an additional number of small follicles, which are not detected sonographically.

Results of hMG treatment in pharmacologic hypogonadotropism

Finally and most importantly we found a significant improvement of pregnancy rates after LHRH-A pretreatment. The pregnancy rate in the hMG/hCG-group was 17% per patient and 5.5% per cycle, in the Buserelin-group 25% per patient and 15% per cycle and in the Decapeptyl-group 25% per patient and 22% per cycle (Table 5). From 740 hMG/hCG cycles without GnRH-A only 66% were sufficient

Table 5. Pregnancy rates of hMG, buserelin/hMG and decapeptyl/hMG-stimulation.

	Number of Patients	Number of Cycle	Pregnancy (n)	Patience (%)	Patience (%)
hMG/hCG	247	740*	41	17	5.5
Buserelin hMG/hCG	233	385	58	25	15
Decapeptyl hMG/hCG	49	55	12	25	22

*Sufficient 66%; premature LH-surge 16%; irreg. LH-fluctuation 18%.

according to the analytical data. In 16% we found a premature LH-discharge and in 18% an irregular LH-fluctuation during stimulation. It is obvious that gonadotropin stimulation during pituitary suppression provokes a more intense ovarian reaction with the respect to the number of follicles as well as the endocrine activity

Incidence of ovarian hyperstimulation syndrome

The ovarian hyperstimulation syndrom (OHS) is still the main side effect of gonadotropin therapy. Therefore it is of interest whether the intensified ovarian response after LHRH/A pretreatment is accompanied by a greater incidence of OSH. Classification of the OSH was done according to Rabau et al [9]. Grade II are patients with abdominal tension, pain, nausea, diarrhea, cystic ovarian enlargement of more than 10 cm and hemoconcentration. The incidence in the hMG/hCG group was 10%, in the Buserelin-group 23% and in the Decapeptyl-group 40%. Grade III of the classification indicates excessively enlarged ovaries with ascites and/or pleural effusion, hypovolemia, hemoconcentration, oligorrhea and hypercoagulability. This was found in the hMG/hCG-group in 0.1%, in the buserelin-group in 0.8% and in the Decapeptyl-group in 5.5%

(Table 7). This means that the combined LHRH-A/hMG-therapy includes a higher pregnancy rate as well as a higher incidence of OSH.

Table 6. Incidence of ovarian hyperstimulation syndrome (OHS) in hMG, buserelin/hMG and decapeptyl/hMG therapy.

OHS	Grade II		Grade III	
hMG/hCG	52	7%	1	0.1%
Buserelin hMG/hCG	89	23%	3	0.8%
Decapeptyl hMG/hCG	22	40%	3	5.5%

CONCLUSIONS

The data demonstrate that induction of pharmacologic hypogonadotropism by prolonged administration of LHRH-A improves ovarian stimulation therapy. Analogue pretreatment reduces LH-levels and prevents pituitary reaction from increasing estrogen activity resulting in an LH surge. The time required for complete pituitary desensitization greatly. Therefore sufficient pituitary suppression has to be proven before starting hMG stimulation. This can be done by measuring the LH fluctuation, by an LHRH test or by performing the E2 provocation-test, which was shown to be the most specific method. The combined use of the LHRH-agonist and hMG reliably excludes an irregular endocrine response during gonadotropin therapy. The response of the patients to hMG stimulation also seems more constant. Moreover, the number of follicles is higher, the functional activity, as measured by the estrogen production, is enhanced and the pregnancy rate is significantly improved. The disadvantage of a higher rate of ovarian hyperstimulation syndrome makes it obligatory to carefully monitor the treatment.

There are also some important practical advantages: ovarian stimulation can be started without any respect to a definite time of bleeding or cycle. Even more important is the much greater flexibility in the timing of hCG administration. Finally it will be in favor of all patients who need ovulation induction, especially oocyte retrieval for IVF or GIFT, because nearly no cycle has to be cancelled. This includes a considerable benefit economically as well as psychologically.

REFERENCES

1. Bettendorf, G and Breckwoldt, M (1964). Klinisch-experimentelle Untersuchungen mit hypophysaerem Human-Gonadotropin. Archiv fuer Gynaekologie, 199, 423

2. Bettendorf, G, Braendle, W, Sprotte, Ch, Poels, W, Lichtenberg, V and Lindner, Ch (1986). Pharmacologic hypogonadotropism - an advantage for hMG-induced follicular-maturation and succeeding fertilization. Horm Metab Res, 18, 656
3. Diczfalusy, E, Johannisson, E, Tillinger, KG and Bettendorf, G (1964). Comparison of the clinical and steroid metabolic effect of human pituitary and urinary gonadotropins in amenorrhoeic women. Acta Endocrinol, 45 (Suppl. 90), 35
4. Bettendorf, G, Braendle, W, Weise, C, Poels, W (1981). Effect of gonadotropin treatment during inhibited pituitary function. In: Insler V and Bettendorf, G (eds.) "Advances in diagnosis and treatment of infertility", p.43 (North Holland: Elsevier)
5. Bettendorf, G, Braendle, W and Sprotte C (1985). Gonadotropin-Stimulation waehrend einer LH/RH-Analogon-induzierten Hemmung der Hypophysenfunktion. Geburstsh u Frauenheilk, 45, 431
6. Lindner, Ch, Braendle, W, Bispink, L, Lichtenberg, V and Bettendorf, G (1987). Gonadotropin-Stimulation und in-vitro-Fertilisation nach selektiver Hypophysen-Suppression durch LH/RH-Analogon. Geburtsch u Frauenheilk, 47, 490
7. Lindner, Ch, Braendle, W, Bispink, L, Lichenberg, V and Bettendorf, G (1987). HMG-induced follicular maturation after blocking of endogenous pituitary gonadotropin discharge. Acta Endocrinol (Copenh.), 283 (Suppl. 114), 169
8. Zimmermann, R, Soor, B, Braendle, W, Lehmann, F, Weise, HC and Bettendorf, G (1982). Gonadotropin therapy of female infertility. Gynecol Obstet Invest, 14, 1
9. Rabau, E, David, A, Serr, DM, Mashiach, S and Lunenfeld, B (1967). Human menopausal gonadotropins for anovulation and sterility. Am J Obstet Gynecol, 98, 92

11

INDUCTION OF OVULATION BY COMBINED GnRH-ANALOGUE/hMG/hCG TREATMENT

M. BRECKWOLDT, F. GEISTHÖVEL, J. NEULEN and H. SCHILLINGER
Department of Obstetrics and Gynecology
Division of Clinical Endocrinology, University of Freiburg
D-7800 Freiburg im Breisgau, FRG

INTRODUCTION

Exogenous administration of human gonadotropins (hMG/hCG) is highly effective in infertility patients suffering from hypogonadotropic amenorrhea classified as WHO I. Pregnancy rates are reported on the order of 80% [1]. In anovulatory infertility patients with normal gonadotropin levels (WHO II), however, hMG/hCG treatment is less effective, achieving pregnancy rates only between 15 and 28% [2].

When superactive GnRH analogues (GnRH-A) became available it was soon recognized that chronic application of these compounds was associated with a desensitization of the pituitary due to prolonged binding of the compound to the GnRH receptor [3]. The desensitization of the pituitary is reflected by a significant suppression of peripheral FSH and LH levels [4, 5]. Chronic application of superactive GnRH-A is responded to by the pituitary by an initial stimulation followed by a phase of progressive pituitary, and consequently gonadal, inhibition. There is also evidence of direct inhibitory effects of GnRH-A at the gonadal level [6].

Based on these findings it was proposed to render infertility patients with normal gonadotropins hypogonadotropic with GnRH-A followed by subsequent stimulation with exogenous gonadotropins to achieve follicular maturation for ovulation induction. Fleming et al [7] reported on 5 infertile women with normal menstrual rhythm but poor luteal phase steroid hormone profiles. These patients were rendered hypogonadotropic with large doses of a GnRH-A and subsequently treated with gonadotropins. Three of these patients conceived.

This paper presents a case report of a patient subjected to GnRH-A/hMG/hCG therapy in order to illustrate the complications that may be associated with this therapeutic approach.

PATIENT

A 31 year old infertility patient is presented. The patient

suffered from anovulatory oligomenorhea due to PCO disease of 6 years duration Basal body temperature (BBT) curves were monophasic. The following peripheral endocrine parameters were determined: FSH, 3.1m U/ml; LH, 8.4 mU/ml; PRL, 6.4 ng/ml and testosterone, 0.9 ng/ml.

Ultrasonography of the ovaries revealed multiple persisting cystic structures.

The patient was treated with clomiphene (100mg/day for 5 days) for several courses followed by biphasic BBT-curves, however, without conception.

Finally the patient was subjected to GnRH-A/hMG/hCG therapy. To achieve pituitary suppression the GnRH-A Decapeptyl® ([D-Trp^6]LHRH, Ferring/Kiel, FRG) was used. Initially the patient received 0.5mg Decapeptyl® daily s.c. followed by i.m. injections of 3.2mg Decapeptyl® in a slow release formulation at 2 week intervals. After complete suppression of ovarian function hMG therapy was initiated at 2 ampoules (150 IU FSH/LH) per day. Ovarian function was monitored by ultrasonography, plasma estradiol (E_2) levels and clinical parameters. On day 9 of the hMG treatment plasma E_2 levels started to rise, on day 12 three leading follicles with a diameter of 20-24mm were detected and several smaller accompanying follicles with a diameter of 14mm. Plasma E_2 levels reached 2800 pg/ml. HCG was injected after the plasma levels of E_2 had dropped to 2400pg/ml. The patient conceived, hyperstimulation was evidenced by cystic enlargement of both ovaries reaching a size of 120x65mm and 120x80mm. At the 8th week of gestation 7 cystic

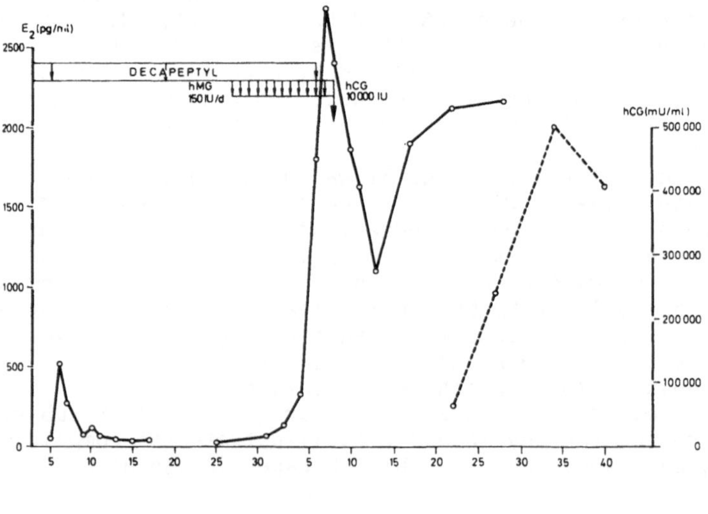

FIGURE 1 Plasma concentrations of estradiol (E_2) and hCG during GnRH-A-hMG/hCG treatment for ovulation induction

structures were detected within the uterine cavity by ultrasonography. Five of these gestational sacs contained single embryos the remaining two contained obviously identical twins. All 9 embryos were vital as evidenced by their heart beats. Plasma hCG levels were found in the order of 500 000 mU/ml.

The treatment course is illustrated in Fig. 1. A sketch of the ultrasonographic finding in the 8th week of gestation is shown in Fig. 2. Within the next two weeks six of the embryos were

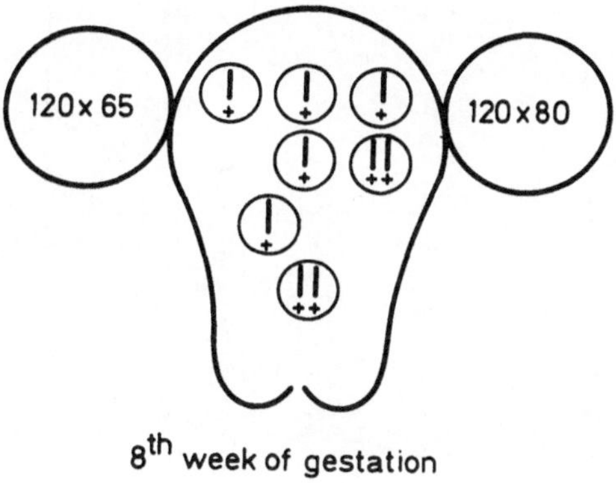

FIGURE 2 Sketch of the ultrasonographic finding at 8 weeks of gestation. Seven intrauterine gestational sacs, 5 with single embryos, 2 with twin embryos. Positive fetal heart beats are indicated by +

eliminated by elective transabdominal puncture at 3 occasions. Figure 3 demonstrates an ultrasonographic detail illustration during puncture, the needle can be visualized within an embryonic bleeding, no further clinical symptoms were recorded. The subsequent course of pregnancy was uneventful. The surviving three fetuses were carried to the 34th week of gestation. Three healthy immature babies were delivered by caesarean section and developed normally.

DISCUSSION

Ovulation induction in patients with polycystic ovarian disease can be achieved by clomiphene or by pulsatile administration of GnRH [8]. However, the prognosis with respect to pregnancy appears to be poor. The suggestion to render these patients

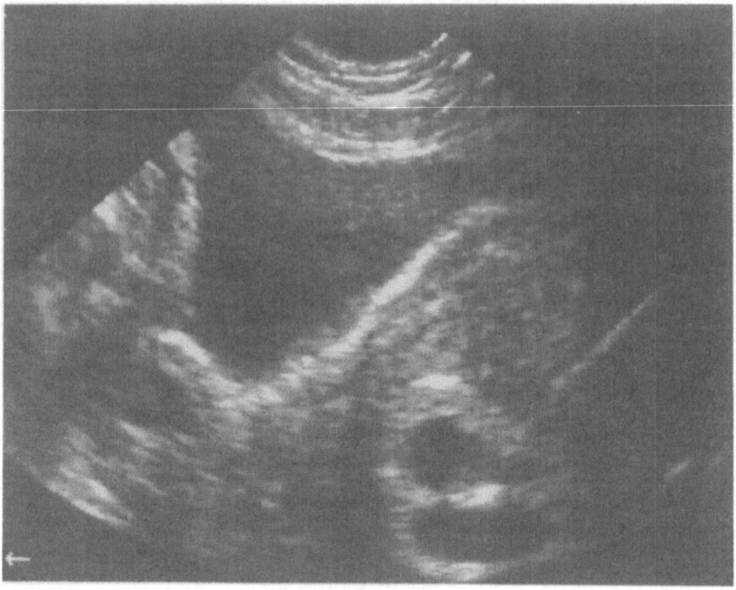

FIGURE 3 Ultrasonographic detail during transabdominal puncture with the needle in situ

hypogonadotropic with subsequent stimulation by hMG may provide a rational approach [9]. Charbonnel et at. [9] described eight clomiphene-resistant PCOD patients treated with a combination of [D-Trp^6]LHRH and hMG/hCG emphasizing the risk of multiple follicular development and ovarian hyperstimulation. The combination of GnRH-A-hMG/hCG has been successfully applied in various IVF-programs with the objective of obtaining a large number of mature follicles and avoiding a premature LH-surge [10, 11, 12]. The recruitment of multiple follicles is obviously associated with this therapeutic regimen. It is well known that PCOD patients are highly susceptible to ovarian hyperstimulation with multiple ovulations and subsequently multiple births after hMG/hCG therapy [2]. The suppression of endogenous gonadotropins by the administration of GnRH-A obviously does not eliminate ovarian hyper-responsiveness in PCOD patients [9, 13]. The patient presented in this communication demonstrates this complication dramatically. Embryo reduction by transabdominal puncture can be regarded as an ultimate solution. The primary goal, of course, should be to avoid multiple conceptions.

REFERENCES

1. Insler. V, and Lunenfeld, B (1983). "Sterilität", p107 (Große Verlag, Berlin)

2 Dor, J, Itzkowic, DJ, Mashiack, S, Lunenfeld, B and Serr, DM (1980). Cumulative conception rates following gonadotropin therapy. Am J Obstet Gynecol, 136, 102

3. Clayton, RN, and Catt, KJ (1979). Receptor binding affinity of gonadotropin-releasing hormone analogs: Analysis by radioligand-receptor assay. Endocrinology, 106, 1154

4. Berquist, C, Nillius, SJ and Wide, L (1979). Inhibition of ovulation in women by intranasal treatment with a luteinizing hormone releasing hormone agonist. Contraception 19, 497

5. Sandow, J (1983). Clinical application of LHRH and its analogues. Clin Endocrinol 18, 571

6. Sharpe, RM (1982). Cellular aspects of the inhibitory actions of LH-RH on the ovary and testis. J Reprod Fert, 64, 517

7. Fleming R, Adam, AH, Barlow, DH, Black, WP, MacNaughton, MC and Coutts JRT (1982). A new systemic treatment for infertility with abnormal hormone profiles. Brit J Obstet Gynaec, 89, 80

8. Schoemaker, J, Burger, CW, van Weissenbruck, MM, Homes, PGA and Eshkol, E (1987). LH-RH and the polycystic ovary. Proc IIIrd. Ann Meet of the Eur Soc Human Reprod and Embryol, p60, (IRL Press, Oxford), Abstract

9. Charbonnel B, Krempf, M. Blanchard, P, Dano, F and Delage, C (1987). Induction of ovulation in polycystic ovary syndrome with a combination of a luteinizing hormone-releasing hormone analog and exogenous gonadotropin. Fertil Steril, 47, 920

10. Porter, RN, Smith, W, Craft, IL, Abdulwahid, NA and Jacobs, HS (1984). Induction of ovulation for in vitro fertlization using Buserelin and gonadotropins. Lancet, 2, 1284

11. Bettendorf, G, Braendle, W and W Sprotte, C (1985). Gonbadotropin-Stimulation während einer LH/RH Analogon-induzierten Hemmung der Hypophysenfunktion. Geburts u Frauenheilk, 45, 431

12. Nader, S, Berkowitz, AS, Maklad, N, Wolf, DP and Held, B (1986). Characteristics of patients with and without gonadotropin surges during follicular recruitment in an in vitro fertilization embryo transfer program. Fertil Steril, 45, 75

13. Fleming, R and Coutts, JRT (1986). Induction of multiple follicular growth in normally menstruating women with endogenous gonadotropin suppression. Fertil Steril, 45, 226

12

COMBINED BUSERELIN AND EXOGENOUS GONADOTROPINS IN OVULATION INDUCTION IN INFERTILE WOMEN WITH NORMAL MENSTRUAL RHYTHM

R. FLEMING, M. CARTER, M.R.P. HAMILTON, M.E. JAMIESON, M.J. HAXTON, W.P. BLACK and J.R.T. COUTTS
University Department of Obstetrics and Gynaecology
Glasgow Royal Infirmary, 10 Alexandra Parade
Glasgow, G31 2ER, Scotland

INTRODUCTION

Infertility amongst women with normal menstrual rhythm, normal pelvic anatomy and normal patterns, is a common and complex clinical problem requiring a comprehensive approach. There are many areas of debate concerning the relative importance of different alleged pathologies and the efficacy of treatments directed at them. It is for these reasons that a strict approach to patient definition and selection should be maintained, although there is no universally adopted systematic approach to either.

The investigation and treatment of patients with oligomenorrhoea, and its intrinsically abnormal ovarian function often associated with polycystic ovary syndrome (PCO) is discussed in the accompanying chapter [1]. This is a group in which the therapeutic role of ovulation induction is understood and established, and the benefits of LH suppression by GnRH agonists (GnRH-A) are clearly demonstrated. However, the situation amongst patients with normal menstrual rhythm, often called "unexplained infertility" is different in that they require a greater intensity of preliminary investigation, and the therapeutic role of ovulation induction is not so widely accepted. It should be noted that many of the "poor responders" described in IVF/GIFT programmes derive from this unexplained group.

The advocacy of ovulation induction in patients with normal menstrual rhythm has 2 limitations. The patients should first demonstrate a pathology of ovarian function derived from abnormal gonadotropin control, and second the therapy must show an efficacy similar to that in patients with primary failure of ovulation due to pituitary failure. Only in this way can the role of abnormal ovarian function in infertility be fully established. The former can only be determined by intensive longitudinal study of reproductive endocrinology and ultrasonography, while the latter requires full clinical control of the ovulation processes.

PATIENTS AND ANALYSES

The patients showed normal menstrual history, had partners with normal semen analyses and laparoscopy revealed normal pelvic anatomy after a primary infertility of at least 3 years. Their investigations were effected by hormonal analyses of plasma samples taken daily from the first week of the cycle until menstruation. The samples were assayed for estradiol (E2), progesterone (P), LH and FSH, using conventional radioimmuno-assays. The patient profiles of these hormones were compared with those of our laboratory normal ranges derived from normal volunteers (n=12) and spontaneous conception cycles (n=8). The most common abnormality revealed by this process was subnormal early luteal phase P profiles following the LH surge [2]. This was defined as the poor P surge (PPS) and was observed in 38% of patients (n=270) [2]. Retained luteal phase cysts were observed in 65% of these cycles. When a series of PPS patients was re-examined using the same protocol in a subsequent cycle 48% showed similar abnormalities. The patients discussed below showed either the PPS profile or no abnormality (unexplained). A second group of PPS patients with minor pelvic complications was also treated with the combined therapy.

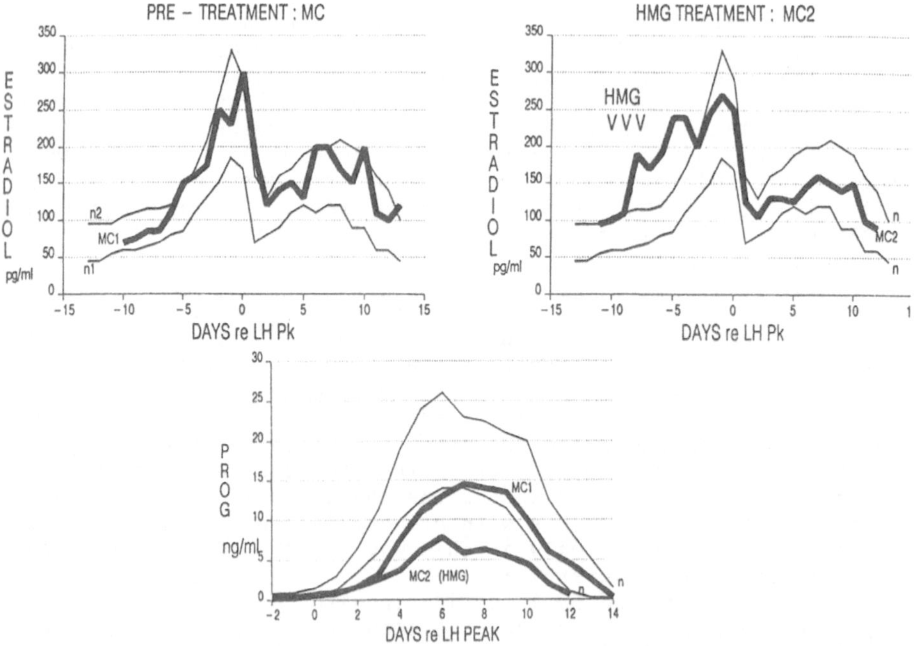

FIGURE 1 E2 and P profiles in a patient in a control cycle and during a cycle treated with exogenous gonadotropins (HMG) in the early follicular phase. Day 0 represents the LH surge as no HCG was administered. The laboratory normal range limits (n) are also shown

PRELIMINARY WORK

It has been postulated that deficient ovarian function may result from a subnormal inter-cycle rise in FSH [3]. Accordingly, human menopausal gonadotropins (HMG; 6 ampoules between days 1 and 6) were administered to a group of infertile women with either normal or subnormal ovarian hormone profiles (unexplained or PPS) in an attempt to improve the early stages of follicular growth. In nearly all cases, there was an increase in follicular growth (raised follicular phase E2) but the subsequent diverse endocrine events were complex, often involving unexpected fluctuations in gonadotropins which resulted in no increase in luteal phase P concentrations, on average, and even no luteinisation at all in some examples. Figure 1 shows an example of one patient whose pretreatment cycle showed normal or near normal profiles, while the treatment cycle demonstrated increased and fluctuating E2 output in combination with reduced luteal phase P concentrations. Profiles such as these can also be observed in patients treated with clomiphene citrate [4]. It was considered that the timing of the LH surge in these cycles was inappropriate to the stage of follicle development, which had been disrupted by the ovarian stimulation.

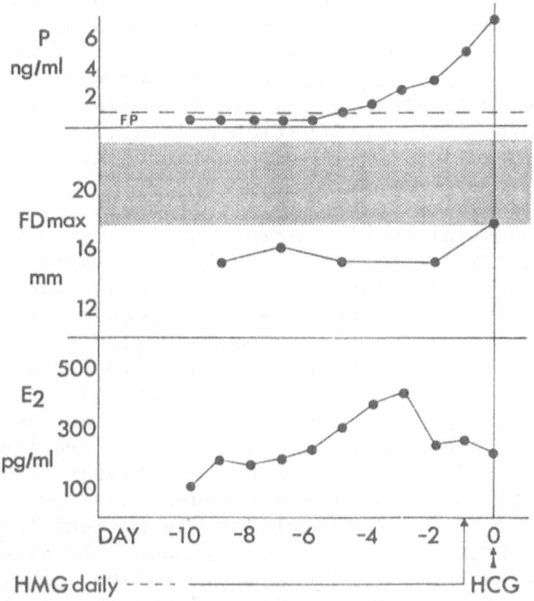

FIGURE 2 P, FDmax (diameter of largest follicle) and E2 profiles in a patient during a cycle treated with HMG (2 amps/day). The HCG was administered (day 0) when the largest follicle reached a diameter of 17mm (mature range lower limit: hatched background). This was after an endogenous LH surge, evidenced by the rise in P concentrations before a mature sized follicle was visualised

When the HMG was administered daily until ultrasound observations identified mature sized follicles (follicle diameter, FD, >17mm) similar events were often observed (Fig. 2), with an LH surge and luteinization occurring before the HCG could be administered. This premature luteinisation was associated with a surge of LH on all occasions, and such responses are rarely encountered in induction of ovulation in women with amenorrhoea due to hypopituitary function. They indicated that the clinical control of the processes of follicular maturation and ovulation in women with normal menstrual rhythm would be facilitated by suppression of endogenous pituitary activity.

USE OF GnRH AND THE COMBINED THERAPY

Protracted administration of GnRH-A was shown to inhibit ovulation in monkeys [5] and in normal women [6], apparently by reduction of circulating LH and FSH concentrations, suggesting that direct clinical control of ovarian function may be possible without interference from endogenous pituitary activity. The first report of the use of GnRH-A to facilitate ovulation induction in women with normal menstrual rhythm [7] was in women showing the PPS abnormality, and effective suppression of both LH and premature luteinisation prior to HCG administration were observed.

The GnRH-A (buserelin, Hoechst UK Ltd.) was administered by intranasal spray (5 x 100μg) starting in the mid-luteal phase of the cycle prior to treatment, and yielded effective suppression of follicular growth after menstruation and until the start of the course of HMG injections which was initiated at clinical convenience.

The HMG injections were administered daily (usually for 7-10 days) after demonstration of ovarian inactivity by estimation of plasma E2 (<80 pg/ml) and by ultrasonic observation of no follicles with FD >9mm. The initial dose was 2 amps/day and this was occasionally modified according to response. HCG was administered when 1-3 follicles of mature size (FD >17mm) were visualised by ultrasonography coincident with plasma E2 concentration consistent with the degree of follicular growth and between 250 and 2500pg/ml. These limits were applied to reduce the risks of multiple conceptions and also of ovarian hyperstimulation. All patients were intensively monitored with plasma E2 estimations (daily) and frequent ovarian ultrasonography. Figure 3 shows an example of one patient through the whole treatment procedure, and clearly shows the absence of a rise in P during the days before HCG administration. Further HCG injections were administered at days +3 and +6 (if the ovaries were not too enlarged) for luteal and endometrial support, although exogenous P would probably suffice in the latter function with the possible benefit of a reduced incidence of hyperstimulation (Smitz, J, Devroey, P and Van Steirtenhem, personal communication, 1987).

GnRH-A therapy was originally discontinued after HCG administration, but the re-initation of therapy in a following cycle, if no pregnancy occurred, became clinically inconvenient, and most patients were thereafter maintained on the GnRH-A therapy until the end of the treatment course (6 cycles or pregnancy).

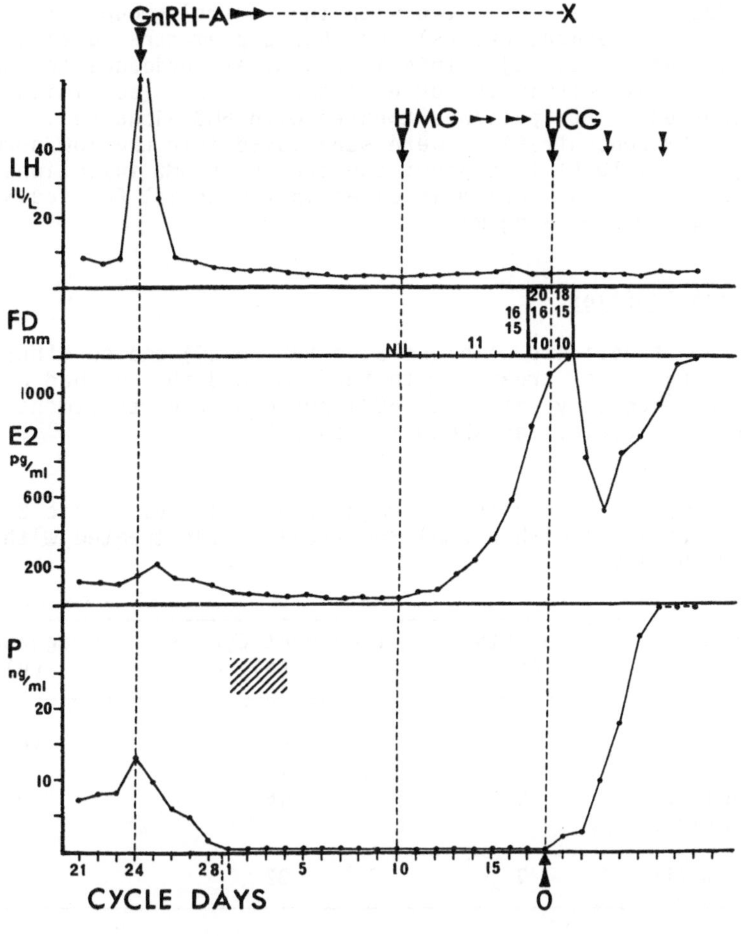

FIGURE 3 E2, P and LH concentrations during the whole combined buserelin (GnRH-A)/HMG/HCG treatment procedure in one patient. The suppression of LH prior to day 0 (HCG administration) resulted in P remaining at follicular phase concentrations through the follicular phase. The striped block represents menstruation after the luteal phase initiation of GnRH-A administration

CLINICAL RESULTS

Premature Luteinization

Observations in a large series of patient cycles (n=84 in 18 patients) treated with the combined therapy showed the effective elimination of premature luteinisation, with a single exceptional patient who required increased doses of the buserelin (1000μg/day). This contrasted with the control group (n=12 patients; 35 treatment cycles) who showed premature luteinization in 40% of the cycles [8]. This is a similar incidence to that observed in patients in IVF or GIFT cycles, and also similar to that recorded in PCO patients treated with HMG alone [9].

The LH concentrations were suppressed into the low/normal range (1.5-6.5 IU/L) throughout the course of HMG injections, and the P concentrations were maintained in the normal follicular phase range (0.25-0.85ng/ml).

Conception Profiles

The series of patients with isolated PPS (n=27) and no other complicating factor treated with the combined therapy had a consistent pregnancy rate (ca. 60%) per course of treatment (maximum of 6 cycles) as shown in Table 1.

Table 1. Clinical results of pregnancies achieved in the 3 groups of patients with normal menstrual rhythm treated with combined therapy.

Patient Group	No. Pts. (n)	Treatment Cycles (n)	Pregnancies (n)
PPS	27	98	16
PPS + Pelvic Complications	9	46	0
No abnormality	7	32	0

Table 1 also shows that patients with unexplained infertility and also those of PPS and a history of pelvic damage (patent Fallopian tubes) yielded no pregnancy, which demonstrates the value of accurate diagnostic procedures.

The cumulative conception rate profile of isolated PPS patients was compared with that of PCO patients treated with the combined therapy [1]. There was a consistently reduced pregnancy rate through the course of treatment, culminating in a pregnancy rate of 60% compared with 80% in the PCO group.

IN VITRO STUDIES OF THOSE FAILING TO CONCEIVE DURING OVULATION INDUCTION

Six patients who have completed a course of ovulation induction

Table 2. Data from studies of PPS patients who have unsuccessfully completed a course of ovulation induction with combined therapy. <RESP represents a subnormal response by reference to the laboratory normal data. The oocyte and embryo scores were subjective assessments made at oocyte collection (based upon degree of cumulus expansion) and at embryo replacement.

Pt. Cycle	Days HMG (n)	Day 0 E2 (ng/ml)	Follicles FD >17 mm (n)	Oocytes (n)	Oocytes Mean Score*	Embryos (n)	Embryos Mean Score*	Note
MP	10	5.5	3	12	3.2	11	7.4	PREG.
MF I	7	8.0	3	9	3.3	1	6	SPERM X
MF II	11	5.9	4	12	3.5	2	6	SPERM X
WB	9	1.1	3	1	3	1	9	<RESP
CM I	12	3.9	0	7	2.8	3	5.8	<RESP
CM II	18	3.0	1	3	2.0	1	5	<RESP
CM III	13	3.8	1	2	2.0	0	-	<RESP
CM IV	16	2.3	0	5	1.5	3	6.9	<RESP
AM I	13	1.8	2	1	3	0	-	<RESP
AM II	12	1.0	2	1	3	1	6	<RESP
DF	15	2.2	3	1	2	-	-	<RESP
Subgroup Average	13.5	2.4	1.5	2.6	2.4	1.3	6.5	
Laboratory Average	11	3.5	4.0	7.0	3.3	3.2	7.5	

*Pregnancies associated exclusively with oocyte scores of 3 and 4, and embryo scores >7.

have been treated in the IVF programme. The multiple follicular development was induced using the same long course combined therapy (HMG administered at 3 or 4 amps/day) and the pre-HCG concentrations of LH and P were identical to those observed during the ovulation induction courses. The oocytes were assessed at laparoscopy and scored according to the degree of cumulus dispersion development, and the embryos were assessed according to the cleavage stage, cell symmetry and fragmentation at replacement (37-66h) after laparoscopic retrieval.

The results (Table 2) show that one patient yielded a large number of oocytes which fertilised and a 3 embryo replacement resulted in a twin pregnancy. It is possible that this patient suffered from undiagnosed tubal problems, while another patient showed a very low fertilisation rate on 2 occasions probably due to the failure of her partner's sperm to "swim up".

The subgroup of 8 cycles in 4 patients on average, showed a consistently subnormal response (<RESP) in all categories analysed. They required more than the average HMG injections and produced lower than average E2 concentrations at HCG administration. There were fewer than the average number of mature follicles and they yielded a reduced number of oocytes and embryos. The quality of the oocytes and embryos were also subnormal. No pregnancy was established in these cycles.

DISCUSSION

It is now well established that the use of a GnRH-A during courses of ovarian stimulation with HMG effectively suppresses LH surges caused by the increased E2. This allows improved clinical control of follicular growth and ovulation, and in the series of patients described above premature (pre-HCG) luteinization was virtually eliminated. This facility has allowed us to study, simultaneously, both the role of abnormal ovarian function in infertility with normal menstrual rhythm and the place in the therapeutic repertoire of controlled ovulation induction in this group of patients.

The clinical results demonstrate sharply that in the absence of a defined abnormality there is no value in ovulation induction. In addition, if there is any history of pelvic damage, which may or may not be related to the endocrine abnormality, then again ovulation induction is redundant.

On the other hand the patients with PPS showed a steady pregnancy rate of 60% in a cycle course with 40% pregnant in 2 courses. This suggests that at least half of the PPS profiles observed are due to abnormal endogenous gonadotropin control of follicular growth and ovulation, since the systematic processes of blockade and replacement of gonadotropins are effective substitutes. This success rate indicates that controlled ovulation induction using the combined therapy has a definite therapeutic role in this specific subgroup of patients.

The first steps towards determining the differences in those patients failing to conceive during the course of ovulation induction have been undertaken with the studies from the IVF programme. The numbers are small at present, but interesting observations are immediately apparent, in that 4 out of 5 patients whose partners showed normal semen motility showed subnormal ovarian responses. Compared with laboratory averages, they showed subnormal ovarian physiological responses in that they required more HMG, and yielded reduced plasma E2 concentratons, as well as fewer mature follicles and oocytes. They also produced oocytes with low qualitative assessment scores and fertilisation. The few embroyos produced also showed a reduced assessment of quality.

It has been argued that reduced oocyte quality and low fertilisation rates derive from increased LH concentrations in the follicular phase [10]. These data demonstrate that this is not the only cause of deficient responses since the LH concentrations were consistently suppressed during these cycles. Therefore, a second group of "poor responders" exists which cannot be improved by LH suppression with combined therapy.

These data suggest that, as with the PCO patients [1], the suppression of endogenous LH and FSH does not substantially alter the basically subnormal ovarian metabolism of these patients. Their responses to exogenous gonadotropins may suffer from the same deficiencies as those apparent during their investigation cycles. Unfortunately, the means to distinguish these patients from those who will conceive on ovulation induction, and possibly in a GIFT programme, are not apparent.

We can summarise that within the patients showing PPS there may be 2 sub-groups presumably related to the origin of the abnormality: those whose PPS derives from abnormal gonadotropin control (the largest group) and therefore amenable to treatment with combined therapy: and the group whose PPS is independent of gonadotropin function and which may be defined as "poor responders".

ACKNOWLEDGEMENTS

The authors wish to thank Dr. P.J. Magill of Hoechst UK Limited for supplies of buserelin

REFERENCES

1. Coutts, JRT, Finnie, S, McNally, W, Conaghan, C, Haxton, MJ, Black, WP, and Fleming, R (1988). Combined buserelin and exogenous gonadotrophin therapy for the treatment of infertility in women with polycystic ovarian disease. Accompanying Chapter, this volume

2. Coutts, JRT (1985). The luteal phase. In Jeffcoate, SL (ed.) "Current Topics in Reproductive Endocrinology". (Chichester: John Wiley and Sons)

3. Ross, GT, Cargille, CM, Lipsett, MB, Rayford, PL, Marshall, JR, Stott, CA and Rodbard, D (1970). Pituitary and gonadal hormones in women during spontaneous and induced ovulatory cycles. Rec Prog Horm Res, 26, 1

4. Fleming, R and Coutts, JRT (1982). Effects of clomiphene treatment on infertile women with normal menstrual rhythm. Brit J Obstet Gynaecol, 89, 749

5. Fraser, HM, Laird, NC and Blakely, DM (1980). Decreased pituitary responsiveness and inhibition of the luteinizing hormone surge and ovulation in the stumptailed monkey (Macaca arctoides) by chronic treatment with an agonist of the luteinizing hormone-releasing hormone. Endocrinology, 106, 452

6. Berquist, C, Nillius, SJ and Wide, L (1979). Inhibition of ovulation in women by intranasal treatment with a luteinizing hormone-releasing hormone agonist. Contraception, 19, 497

7. Fleming, R, Adams, AH, Barlow, DH, Black, WP, Macnaughton, MC and Coutts, JRT (1982). A new systematic treatment for infertile women with abnormal hormone profiles. Brit J Obstet Gynaecol, 80, 80

8. Fleming, R and Coutts, JRT (1986). Induction of multiple follicular growth in normally menstruating women with endogenous gonadotropin suppression. Fertil Steril, 45, 226

9. Fleming, R, Yates, RWS, Haxton, MJ, Coutts, JRT, Hamilton, MPR and Conaghan, C (1987). Ovulation induction using the combination of buserelin and exogenous gonadotrophins in women with functional pituitaries. Brit J Clin Practice, 41, (Suppl No 48), 34

10. Stanger, JD and Yovich, JL (1985). Reduced in vitro fertilization of human oocytes from patients with raised basal luteinizing hormone levels during the follicular phase. Brit J Obstet Gynaecol, 92, 385

13

COMBINED BUSERELIN AND EXOGENOUS GONADOTROPHIN THERAPY FOR THE TREATMENT OF INFERTILITY IN WOMEN WITH POLYCYSTIC OVARIAN DISEASE

J.R.T. COUTTS, S. FINNIE, W. McNALLY, C. CONAGHAN, M.J. HAXTON, W.P. BLACK and R. FLEMING
University Department of Obstetrics and Gynaecology
Glasgow Royal Infirmary, 10 Alexandra Parade
Glasgow G31 2ER, Scotland

INTRODUCTION

A considerable proportion of the women who attend infertility clinics menstruate but do not show normal menstrual rhythm. Oligomenorrhea (menstrual cycles occurring at >6 week intervals) was found in 16% of 1,162 new patients attending the Infertility Clinic at Glasgow Royal Infirmary during the years 1975-1983 [1]. The exact status of such patients with respect to ovarian function is difficult to assess since menstruation, when it occurs, although obviously a response to hormone withdrawal may or may not be associated with a preceding ovulation. In this chapter the results of in-depth investigations on 55 infertile women with oligomenorrhea are presented.

Polycystic ovarian disease (PCO) is a condition which was first described by Stein and Leventhal in 1935 [2]. It is a badly defined disease syndrome in which the women usually have oligomenorrhea and elevated plasma luteinising hormone (LH) concentrations. Such patients may or may not also have elevated plasma androgen concentrations, raised plasma oestrone to oestradiol ratios, and may or may not be hirsute and/or obese. In recent years ovarian ultrasound scans have also been used to describe PCO [3] but since such descriptions have been often associated with normal menstrual rhythm it is unlikely that all of these definitions are describing a homogeneous group of women. As a result of poor definitions it has become increasingly difficult to compare the results of different treatment regimes for PCO since the patient groups treated often differ. However, it is possible to generalise with regard to such treatments. This chapter also describes the use of combined buserelin and exogenous gonadotrophins (HMG and HCG) for ovulation induction in PCO patients (oligomenorrheic patients with elevated circulating LH concentrations).

OVARIAN PHYSIOLOGY IN PATIENTS WITH PRIMARY OLIGOMENORRHEA

Patients and methods

Fifty-five patients with oligomenorrhea (cycle length >6 weeks) and husbands whose semenology was acceptable in terms of both quality and quantity were investigated. All of these women had previously been treated for at least 12 months with clomiphene citrate (up to 250mg per cycle) without achieving pregnancy. Each patient was investigated and monitored as described in Figure 1.

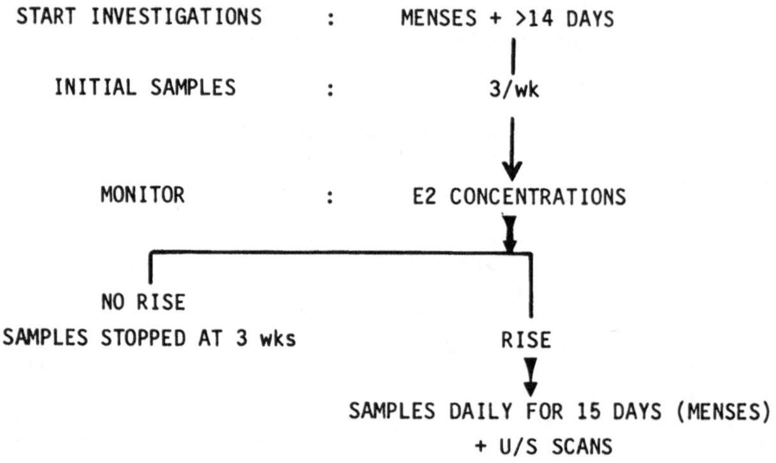

FIGURE 1 Oligomenorrhea and Infertility Investigation Protocol

Three plasma samples per week were provided for a minimum of 3 weeks beginning at least 14 days after the onset of menstruation. Samples on receipt were immediately assayed to determine the levels of circulating oestradiol. Where no oestradiol rise was observed sampling was terminated after 3 weeks whereas when an oestradiol rise, indicative of ovarian activity, was observed patients were immediately changed to a daily sampling procedure. Daily samples were collected for at least 14 days or until the onset of menstruation. All patients had basal ovarian ultrasound scans performed at initiation of therapy and, where ovarian activity was observed, sequential ovarian ultrasound scans were performed to monitor any follicular growth.

The plasma concentrations of LH, follicle stimulating hormone (FSH), oestradiol (E2), oestrone (E1) and androstenedione (A) were determined in all samples using sensitive specific radioimmunoassays and the plasma progesterone (P) concentrations were determined using a sensitive specific radioimmunoassay in all samples after evidence of ovarian activity had been obtained.

RESULTS

Figure 2 shows the mean LH concentrations in the 55 patients: 71% showed elevated basal LH concentrations, 5% showed high/normal

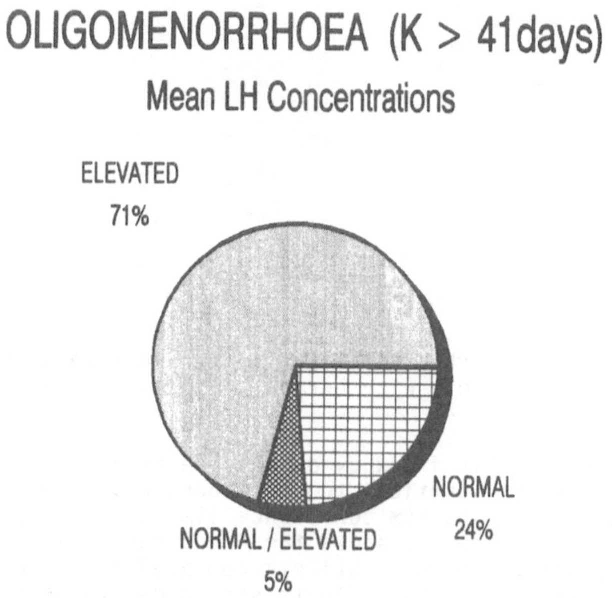

FIGURE 2 Oligomenorrhea and infertility: mean LH concentrations (n=55 patients)

basal LH levels, whilst 24% showed normal LH levels. Figure 3 shows the incidence of follicle growth as monitored by both E2 concentrations and ovarian ultrasound in the patients with high and normal LH levels. In both groups of patients approximately 50% showed evidence of follicular growth and this incidence was not affected by the basal LH level. Ovulation as monitored by E2 and ovarian ultrasound apparently occurred in 25/55 patients. Plasma P concentrations were used to construct a P index (Figure 4) for the post-ovulatory phase in the patients with apparent ovulation by comparison with laboratory values from fertile

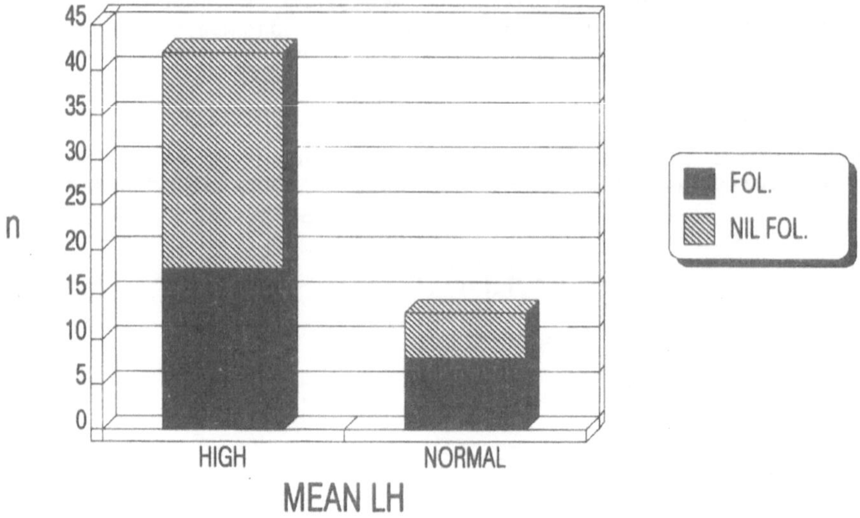

FIGURE 3 Oligomenorrhea and infertility: incidence of follicular growth in patients with normal and elevated LH levels

volunteers [4]. This index by definition is 100 where the patient concentrations are identical to the laboratory normal mean concentrations and the 95% confidence limits of normal values are from 70 to 130. Figure 5 shows the P indices of all of the "ovulatory" oligomenorrhea patients compared to the normal values. Twenty of the 25 patients showed deficient luteal phases similar to the poor P surge (PPS) group described in women with normal menstrual rhythm [5] and whose treatment is described in the accompanying chapter [4]. As was the case with follicular growth, the P index was apparently unaffected by the basal LH concentrations. The occurrence of these deficient luteal phases raises doubts as to whether satisfactory ovulation actually had occurred [6].

From these investigations we conclude that primary oligomenorrheic women are infertile for two reasons: 1) ovulation was a relatively rare event and 2) where ovulation occurred it was usually deficient or at least was accompanied by a deficient luteal phase. These ovulation problems did not appear to be related to the basal circulating concentrations of LH.

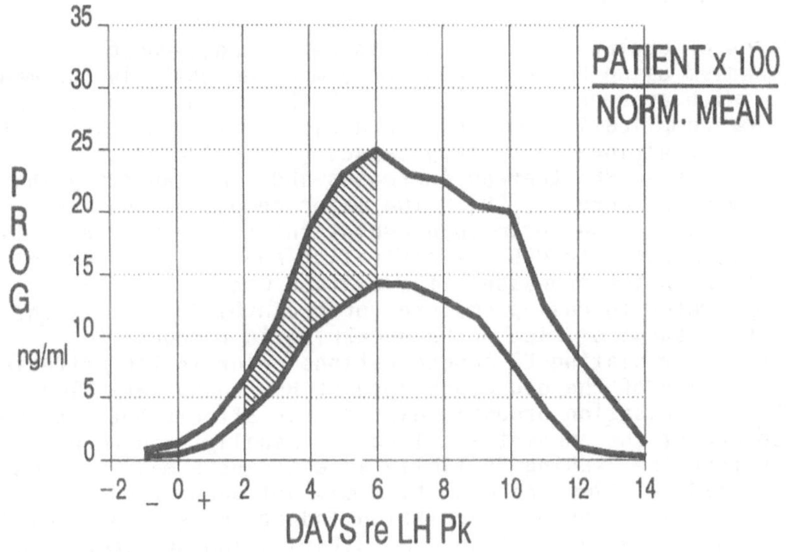

FIGURE 4 The Progesterone Index - Definition

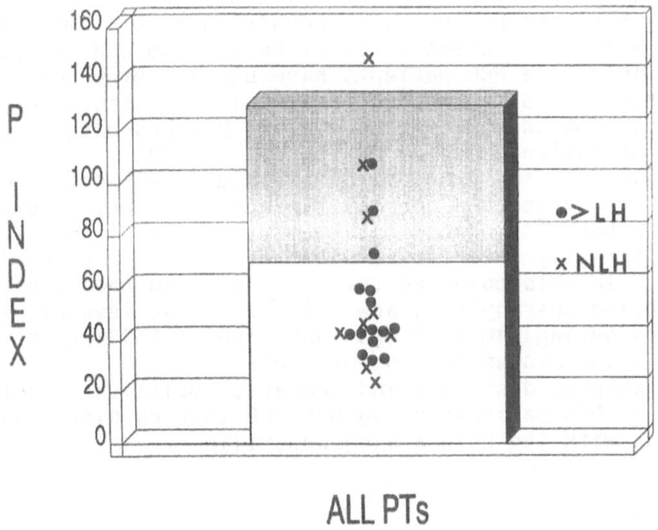

FIGURE 5 Oligomenorrhea and Infertility: progesterone indices in apparently ovulatory patients. Comparison of patients with elevated LH (Δ) with those with normal LH(x) levels. Hatched background = normal fertile range for P

INDUCTION OF OVULATION

Induction of ovulation in women with hypogonadotrophic hypogonadism using HMG has been performed successfully for many years. With appropriate monitoring, both a high pregnancy rate and a low complication rate can be achieved [7]. However, with increasing functional pituitary capacity, the incidence of complications in HMG therapy increases and simultaneously the pregnancy rate decreases [8]. The major complications are hyperstimulation and "premature ovulation" [9]. The former is usually a response to HCG administration and as such does not interfere with the processes of ovulation whereas the latter, which we prefer to call premature (or pre-HCG) luteinisation, is caused by a surge or rise of LH occurring in response to increasing circulating E2 concentrations prior to the criteria for administration of the ovulatory dose of HCG being satisfied. This pre-HCG luteinisation probably has adverse effects both at the ovarian and at the endometrial levels. Usually such LH rises occur before the leading follicle has achieved a mean follicular diameter (FD) of 17mm and ovulation may not occur [10].

The patients for whom ovulation induction is being considered in this chapter have functional pituitaries and are therefore a high risk group for the occurrence of pre-HCG luteinisation.

OVULATION INDUCTION IN WOMEN WITH PCO

The first line treatment for infertile patients with PCO is anti-oestrogen therapy, using compounds such as clomiphene citrate and shows variable success rates of between 30 and 40% [11]. The remaining infertile PCO patients have usually proceeded to HMG/HCG therapy which, despite the problematical side effects of hyperstimulation and "premature ovulation", has also resulted in 30 to 40% of patients achieving conception [12].

To alleviate the problems of pre-HCG luteinisation which compromise ovulation and correct timing of coitus, a combined therapy has been introduced to attempt to prevent endogenous pituitary activity interfering with the induction of ovulation processes. In this combined therapy the antigonadotrophic effects of LHRH analog therapy [13] are utilised to achieve pituitary suppression during simultaneous induction of follicular growth and ovulation using exogenous gonadotrophins.

This chapter describes and compares ovulation induction therapies in PCO patients using HMG/HCG therapy alone and in combination with the LHRH analog buserelin.

PATIENTS

Women with oligomenorrhea who showed typical biochemical/endocrinological characteristics of PCO (elevated plasma LH, elevated plasma LH/FSH ratios) were treated in this study. Most of these patients had confirmed polycystic ovaries by ovarian ultrasound and/or ovarian biopsy. All of these PCO women had been infertile for a minimum of 3 years, had husbands whose semenology was acceptable in terms of both quality and quantity and had been treated unsuccessfully (in terms of pregnancies) with clomiphene citrate in varying doses (up to 250mg x 5/cycle) for at least 12 cycles.

TREATMENT REGIMENS

Patients were treated using either HMG/HCG therapy alone or HMG/HCG therapy after and during continued pituitary suppression with the LHRH analog.

LHRH Analog Therapy

In PCO patients LHRH analog therapy was initiated randomly after plasma E2 and P concentrations and ovarian ultrasound had confirmed that the patient was not either about to ovulate or in the luteal phase. If the patient was either immediately pre or post ovulatory initiation of buserelin therapy was not commenced days until 4 or more days after the ensuing menses. The buserelin therapy was initiated using a daily dose of 500µg intranasally (100µg at each of 07.00, 11.00, 15.00, 19.00 and 23.00 h). In most patients the initial stimulatory effect of the LHRH analog therapy was sufficient to elicit some ovarian activity which resulted in a withdrawal bleed within 7 to 14 days. Whereas pituitary suppression was established in women with normal menstrual rhythm by the fifth day after initiation of buserelin [14] PCO patients' LH levels did not reach basal normal cycle levels until up to 14 days of treatment (Figure 6). The occurrence of the withdrawal bleed after initiation of LHRH analog therapy was a good monitor of when a hypogonadotrophic hypogonadal state had been achieved. Once this state had been achieved and confirmed by low plasma E2 concentrations and lack of follicular growth by ovarian ultrasound the period of induced hypogonadism could be extended for patient or clinical convenience prior to commencing the induction of ovulation procedures. LHRH therapy continued throughout successive ovulation induction procedures at the daily dosage described above until pregnancy was established or the treatment course was terminated (6 treatment cycles).

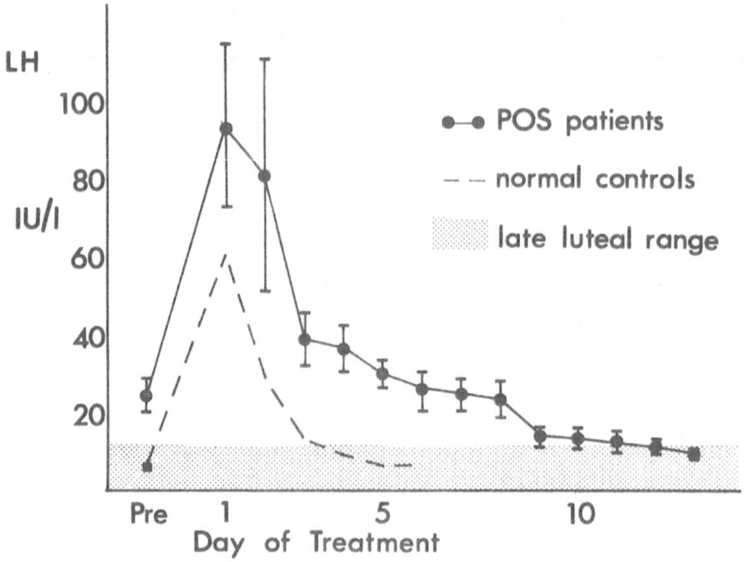

FIGURE 6 Mean plasma LH concentrations in response to initiation of buserelin treatment (500μg/day) in patients with PCO compared to those in patients with normal menstrual rhythm. Note the elevated starting levels in the PCO patients and the fact that suppression to basal levels (hatched background) did not occur until at least 12 days of treatment

<u>Ovulation Induction</u>

Follicular growth and induction of ovulation were induced in both therapy groups using the same regimen. This involved daily injections of HMG until day 0 criteria were achieved when 5,000 IU HCG (day 0) were administered. In the case of HMG/HCG therapy alone injections of HMG were initiated randomly in the oligomenorrheic cycles after confirmation, by plasma E2 concentrations and ovarian ultrasound scans, that no ovarian follicular activity was present. Alternatively, injections of HMG were initiated 4 days after the onset of menses where appropriate. In the case of the combined LHRH analog/HMG/HCG therapy HMG injections were initiated after induction of

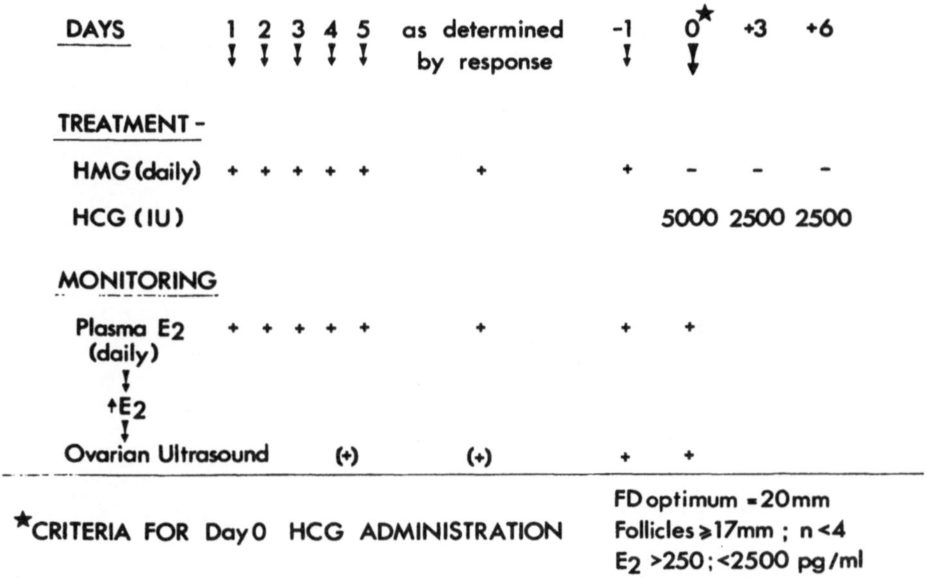

FIGURE 7 Standard protocol for ovulation induction using HMG/HCG therapy

hypogonadotrophic hypogonadism when appropriate as described above. The initial dose of Pergonal was 2 amps (150 IU FSH; 150 IU LH) daily i.m. and each patient's dose was titrated dependent upon her response. Responses to treatment were monitored daily using a rapid (2 h) plasma E2 radioimmunoassay and serial ovarian ultrasound scans were performed when plasma E2 concentratons indicated they were appropriate. In retrospect plasma P concentrations over the last few days leading up to day 0 were determined to assess the occurrence of pre-HCG luteinisation which was deemed to have occurred if plasma P concentrations rose to 1.5ng/ml or more prior to HCG administration. Day 0 criteria for HCG administration were <4 follicles of follicular diameter >17mm in the presence of E2 concentrations appropriate for the total follicular volume present and >250pg/ml and <2,500pg/ml. All patients received luteal luteal support injections of 2,500 IU HCG on days +3 and +6 unless ovarian ultrasound scans on +6 showed excessive ovarian enlargement.

Figure 7 shows the ovulation induction regimen used for both HMG/HCG therapy alone and for the combined therapy after production of hypogonadotrophic hypogonadism whilst Figure 8 depicts the complete combined Buserelin/HMG/HCG therapy in one patient.

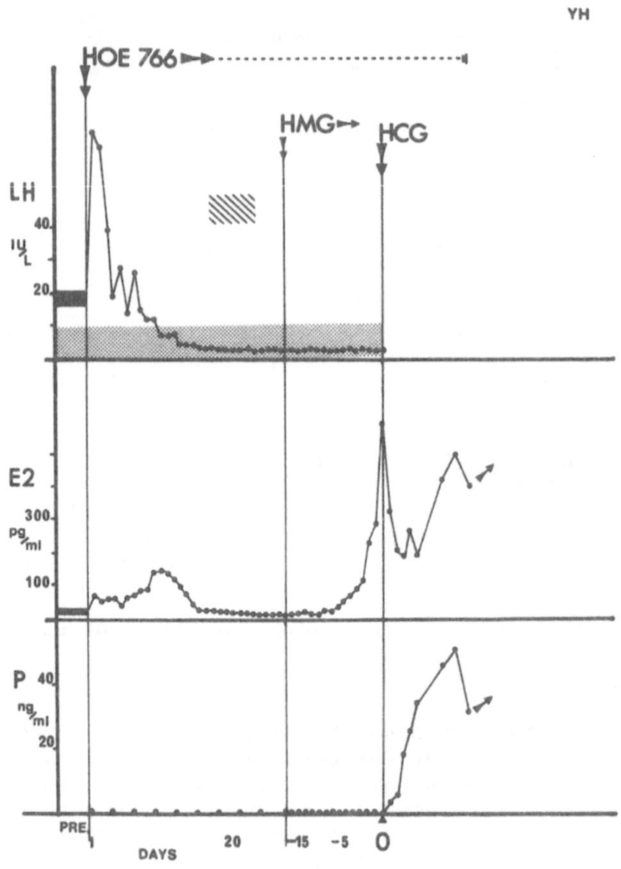

FIGURE 8 Protocol for combined buserelin (GnRH)/HMG/HCG ovulation induction in a woman with PCO. Buserelin is initiated randomly in the cycles (often anovulatory) and HMG injections are commenced at least 14 days later. This particular patient conceived a singleton pregnancy during this treatment

RESULTS

Table 1 lists the complete clinical results of the use of the two treatment regimes in PCO patients. Thirty-eight per cent of these

Table 1. Comparison in PCO patients of results following ovulation induction using hMG/hCG alone and in combination with buserelin.

Therapy	Patients (n)	Treatment Cycles (n)	Patients with Pre-hCG Luteinization (n)	(% Patients)	Pregnancies (n)	(% Patients)
hMG/hCG	45	120	15	33	19	38
Buserelin/ hMG/hCG	38	102	0	0	30	79

patients achieved pregnancy using HMG/HCG alone [15] but with this regimen one-third of the patients treated showed pre-HCG luteinisation. By contrast pre-HCG luteinisation was completely eliminated during the combined therapy and a significantly increased pregnancy rate (79%) was achieved.

Patients who showed pre-HCG luteinisation on HMG/HCG alone and who did not become pregnant were treated subsequently with the combined therapy. Figure 9 shows the LH and P profiles during the 5 days prior to HCG administration (day 0) in the same patients during treatment with HMG/HCG alone and in combination with buserelin. In the HMG/HCG alone cycles significant rises in LH and consequently in plasma P concentrations were observed during this period whereas such pre-HCG luteinisation was completely eliminated by the combined therapy. Thus, during combined LHRH analog/HMG/HCG therapy complete clinical control of the processes of ovulation was possible without interference from endogenous pituitary activity, and a high pregnancy rate resulted. Figure 10 shows the cumulative pregnancy rate for PCO patients up to 6 cycles of combined therapy. Sixty per cent of patients achieved pregnancy by 4 months of therapy and 80% by the completion of 6 treatment cycles.

Apart from pre-HCG luteinisation the other main complication of HMG/HCG therapy alone is the occurrence of hyperstimulation or over-responsiveness [8]. Figure 11 shows the total number of small (10-13.9mm), medium (14.0-16.9mm) and large (>17mm) follicles present on days -5, -3 and during the 24 h prior to day 0 HCG administration in the ovaries of the same patients treated respectively with HMG/HCG alone and the combined therapy. There was no significant difference between the numbers of follicles of all sizes present on the two forms of treatment showing that the responsiveness of the polycystic ovaries was unaffected by suppressing the basal plasma LH concentrations.

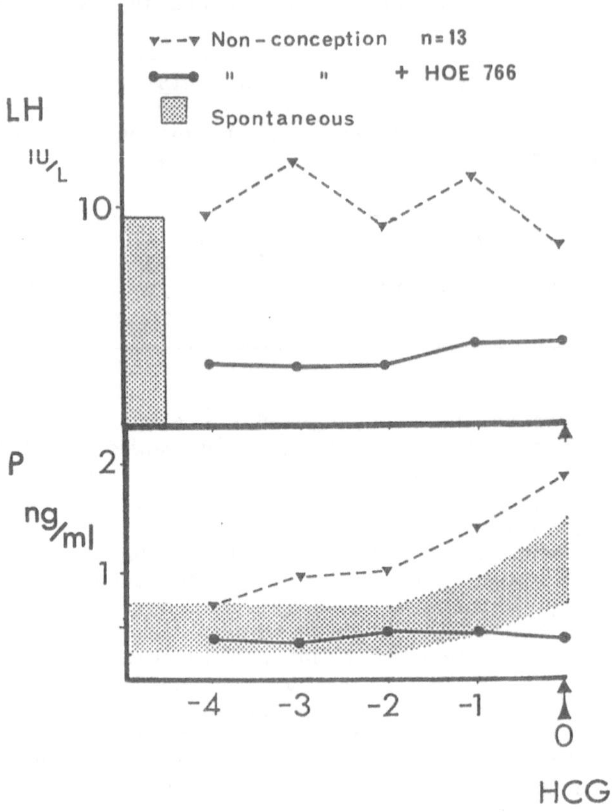

FIGURE 9 Mean LH and progesterone (P) profiles during the five days prior to HCG administration (day 0) in the same group of PCO patients treated for ovulation induction with either HMG/HCG (HMG) or combined buserelin/HMG/HCG. Pre-HCG elevations in LH and consequential pre-HCG luteinisation were observed on HMG/HCG therapy whereas the combined therapy completely eliminated these phenomena

DISCUSSION

First-line treatment for infertile women with PCO clomiphene citrate therapy results in pregnancy rates of between 30 and 40 per cent. The results presented in this study confirmed that of the failures to achieve pregnancy using anti-estrogens

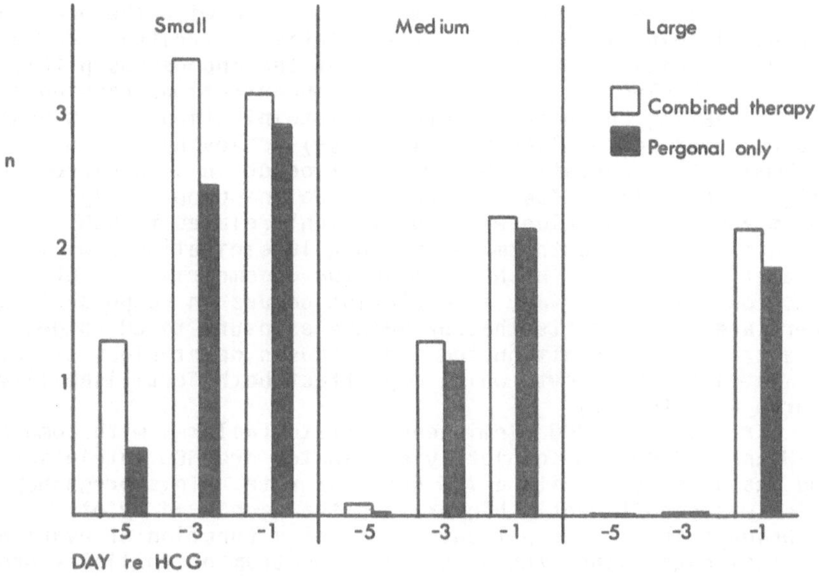

FIGURE 10 Cumulative conception rate through 6 cycles in women with PCO treated with combined buserelin/HMG/HCG for ovulation induction

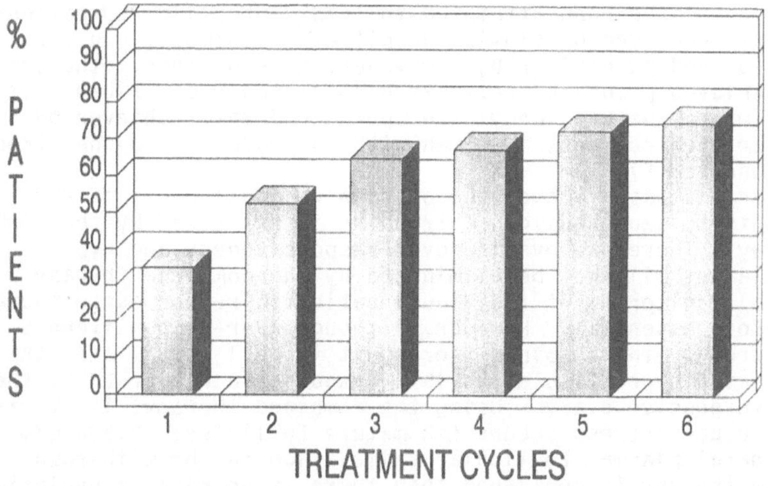

FIGURE 11 Comparison of the mean numbers of small (10-13.9mm), medium (14-16.9mm) and large >17mm) follicles visualised by ultrasound on days -5, -3 and -1 [during the 24 h prior to HCG (day 0)] in the same patients treated for ovulation induction with both HMG/HCG alone (HMG) and buserelin/HMG/HCG (combined) therapies

approximately a further 40% became pregnant using HMG/HCG alone. This latter therapy, however, was associated with the occurence of pre-HCG luteinisation in 33% of the patients treated. These pre-HCG luteinisation is a function of the endogenous pituitary response to elevated circulating E2 concentrations causing a rise in circulating LH which effects the luteinisation. This usually occurs prior to the leading follicle(s) achieving a mature size (>17mm) [16]. Ovulation may well not occur in such circumstances [10] and even if it does coitus will be inappropriately recommended to coincide with "ovulation" related to HCG administration. Furthermore, pre-HCG luteinisation P will produce endometrial changes which may make the endometrium out of synchrony with the ovary if ovulation occurs in response to HCG. There are also reports that premature exposure to LH surges (even of a transient and attenuated type) causes deleterious effects at the level of the oocyte which may effect both fertilisability and embryo quality [17].

Treatment of PCO clomiphene citrate failures with combined LHRH analog/HMG/HCG completely eliminated pre-HCG luteinisation and was associated with a 79% pregnant rate. This pregnancy rate, which was significantly higher than that achieved by other techniques in similar patients, was not a function of ovarian responsiveness since the number and spectrum of follicles grown was identical on both HMG/HCG alone and on combined therapy. The high pregnancy rate achieved by the combined therapy could therefore be directly attributed to the elimination of pre-HCG luteinisation ensuring that endometrial and ovarian activities were in synchrony, that coitus was properly timed and that any oocytes released were of as high a quality as possible. Other treatments have been attempted to treat infertile PCO patients who had not conceived on clomiphene citrate treatment, e.g., pulsatile LHRH [3] and pure FSH [18]. However, none of these other methods has achieved pregnancy rates as high as those described in this study where the pregnancy rate approached that achieved by appropriate treatment in women with idiopathic hypogonadotrophic hypogonadism [7].

As discussed above, the ovarian responsiveness of PCO patients to exogenous gonadotrophins is unaltered by the combined therapy. Therefore ovarian over-responsiveness and hyper-stimulation will not be eliminated by the combined therapy. Careful monitoring of individual patients' responses to therapy is therefore essential. However, although over-responsiveness is unaltered by the combined therapy it is well established that the associated hyperstimulation is a response to HCG or LH by the over-responsive ovary. Using the combined therapy, if ovarian over-responsiveness occurs (>3 mature follicles; >2,500pg/ml E2/ml peripheral plasma) follicular stimulation can be withdrawn. If analog therapy is continued then there is no risk of ovulation occurring since endogenous LH surges are eliminated and hence both multiple pregnancy and/or hyper-stimulation will not occur. After an appropriate time, when plasma E2 concentrations have returned to basal levels and ovarian cystic structures are not visualisable by ultrasound, follicular stimulation can be reinitiated and a further course of ovulation induction therapy performed.

The results of combined buserelin/HMG/HCG therapy for infertile women with PCO presented in this chapter indicate that such treatments should become at least second line treatment (after anti-oestrogen successes have been removed). Indeed, only economic reasons (drug and monitoring costs) would prevent it becoming the first line therapy for infertile women with PCO.

REFERENCES

1. Haxton, MJ and Black, WP (1987). The aetiology of infertility in 1,162 investigated couples. Clin Exper Obstet Gynaecol, XIV, 75
2. Stein, IF and Leventhal, ML (1935). Amenorrhea associated with bilateral polycystic ovaries. Am J Obstet Gynecol, 29, 181
3. Jacobs, HS, Adams, J, Franks, S, Kelly, C, Mason, WP, Morris, DV, Ross, L, Sutherland, R, Chambers, GR and van der Spuy, ZM (1984). Induction of ovulation with LHRH - problems, indications and contra-indications. In: Labrie, F, Belanger, A and Dupont, A (eds.) "LHRH and its Analogues - Basic and Clinical Aspects". p.464. (Amsterdam: Elsevier Science Publishers B.V.)
4. Fleming, R, Carter, M, Hamilton, MPR, Jamieson, ME, Haxton, MJ, Black, WP and Coutts, JRT (1988). Combined Buserelin and exogenous gonadotrophins (HMG, HCG) in ovulation induction in infertile women with normal menstrual rhythm. Accompanying Chapter.
5. Coutts, JRT (1985). The deficient luteal phase, In: Jeffcoate, SL (ed.) "The Luteal Phase". p.101. (Chichester: John Wiley and Sons)
6. Coutts, JRT, Adam, AH and Fleming, R (1982). The deficient luteal phase may represent an anovulatory cycle. Clin Endocrinol, 17, 389
7. Fleming, R, Coutts, JRT and Hamilton, MPR (1984). Evidence against genetic factors causing major loss of embryos. Brit Med J, 288, 1576
8. Lunenfeld, B and Insler, V eds (1978). "Infertility" (Berlin: Grosse Verlag)
9. Gemzell, CA, Kenman, E and Jones, JR (1978). Premature ovulation during administration of human menopausal gonadotropins in non-ovulatory women. Infertility, 1, 1
10. Stanger, JD and Yovich, JL (1984). Failure of human oocyte release at ovulation. Fertil Steril, 41, 827
11. MacGregor, AH, Johnson, JE and Bundle, CA (1968). Further clinical experience with clomiphene citrate. Fertil Steril, 19, 616
12. Wang, CF and Gemzell, CA (1980). The use of human gonadotropins for the induction of ovulation in women with polycystic ovary disease. Fertil Steril, 33, 479
13. Bergquist, C, Nillius, SJ and Wide, L (1979). Inhibition of ovulation in women by intranasal treatment with a luteinising hormone releasing hormone agonist. Contraception, 19, 479

14. Fleming, R, Adams, AH, Barlow, DH, Black, WP, Macnaughton, MC and Coutts, JRT (1982). A new systematic treatment for infertile women with abnormal hormone profiles. Brit J Obstet Gynaecol, 80, 80
15. Diamond, MP and Wentz, AC (1986). Ovulation induction with human menopausal gonadotropins. Obstet Gynaecol Surv, 40, 480
16. Hackeloer, BJ, Fleming R, Robinson, HP, Adam, AH and Coutts, JRT (1978). Correlation of ultrasonic and endocrinologic assessment of follicular development. Am J Obstet Gynecol, 135, 122
17. Stanger, JD and Yovich, JL (1985). Reduced in vitro fertilisation of human oocytes from patients with raised basal luteinising hormone levels during the follicular phase. Brit J Obstet Gynaecol, 92, 385
18. Venturoli, S, Fabbri, R, Paradisi, R, Magrini, O, Porcu, E, Orsini, LF and Flamigni, C (1983). Induction of ovulation with human urinary follicle-stimulating hormone: endocrine pattern and ultrasound monitoring. Eur J Obstet Gynaecol Reprod Biol, 16, 135

14

COMPARISON BETWEEN SHORT AND LONG PROTOCOLS USING A COMBINATION OF LHRH AGONIST AND GONADOTROPINS

L. METTLER
Department of Obstetrics and Gynecology
University of Kiel, 2300 Kiel, FRG

INTRODUCTION

As good success rates in human IVF and FIGT/ET at the present time require multiple follicular maturation and the transfer of multiple fertilized oocytes or embryos, methods to improve homogeneous oocyte maturation and resulting in a larger number of embryos to be transferred would be invaluable [1].

The majority of IVF and GIFT/ET programs use clomiphene, clomiphene plus menopausal gonadotropins, or even pure gonadotropin stimulation for stimulation of cycles. We know that in several cases interruption of preovulatory follicular maturation occurs as a consequence of premature LH surges [2, 3]. The occurrence of such LH surges in most cases prevents the successful treatment of patients. Investigations in monkeys have demonstrated that the constant infusion of GnRH suppresses the secretion of hypophysial gonadotropins [4, 5]. Agonist analogues of LHRH impede LH surges through a down-regulation of the hypophysial-gonadal axis. We have applied this principle therefore to block premature gonadotropin secretion using a potent LHRH agonist synthesized by Schally and co-workers [6].

In the present paper we describe this new method of multifollicular maturation using the LHRH agonist [D-Trp^6]LHRH (decapeptyl) with consecutive gonadotropin stimulation. Two methods applying decapeptyl and FSH or HMG resulted for use in patients requiring follicular puncture, IVF and ET.

MATERIAL AND METHODS

Sixty-seven patients, their ages ranging from 32 to 40 years, from the IVF/ET and GIFT program of Kiel University Hospital were included in this study. In all of them premature LH rises occurred during previous stimulations with HMG/HCG. Down regulation was performed using decapeptyl supplied by Ferring [Kiel, W. Germany] with subcutaneous injections of 500µg and 100µg. The patients were divided into two groups. Individualised FSH or HMG stimulations were started on the second day of the cycle according to the oestradiol reaction of the patient.

GROUP 1

Decapeptyl, 500µg daily subcutaneously, was administered starting directly after ovulation, at the beginning of the luteal phase, until there was evidence of exhaustion of the pituitary reaction to a GnRH test. This was followed by further administration of 100µg decapeptyl daily along with HMG or FSH.

GROUP 2

Along with HMG or FSH stimulation, decapeptyl was administered at 500µg daily from the second to the seventh day of the cycle and then the dose was reduced to 100µg daily.

During stimulation with HMG or FSH, daily serum estimations of LH, FSH, and oestradiol were performed; HCG was administered when the criteria of sufficient follicular maturity were obtained [1]. The last injection of decapeptyl was given on the day of HCG administration. Thirtysix hours after HCG administration, vaginosonographically guided follicular punctures were performed [7]. All of the recovered oocytes were inseminated with the husband's sperms, examined after 16 hours for pronuclei formation, and after 48 hours for the stage of division reached. All embryos, developing from oocytes with 2 pronuclei, were transferred back into the uterine cavity of the patient.

Table I. In vitro fertilization at the Department of Obstetrics and Gynecology University of Kiel in the Years 1982 - 1987.

Year	FP	Oozytes		Transfers		Embryos		Pregnancies			Delivered Babies
	n	n	$\bar{x}$	n	% Per FP	n	$\bar{x}$	n	% Per FP	% Per Transf.	
1982	140	210	1.5	70	50.0	110	1.6	4	2.9	5.7	-
1983	153	430	2.8	95	62.1	191	2.0	8	5.2	8.4	6
1984	119	462	3.9	78	65.6	202	1.6	18	15.1	23.1	12
1985	177	1,049	5.9	142	80.2	418	2.9	36	20.3	25.4	18
1986	169	1,206	7.1	152	89.9	550	3.6	43	25.4	28.3	43
1987	310	2,036	6.6	253	81.6	905	3.6	71	22.9	28.1	66
Σ	1,068	5,393	4.6	790	71.6	2,322	2.5	180	15.2	19.8	145

RESULTS

In the years 1982 to 1987 in Kiel an increasing number of patients were subjected to follicular puncture aiming at oocyte recovery, IVF and ET. Table 1 shows the number of follicular punctures performed, the absolute number of pregnancies achieved (excluding chemical pregnancies), the pregnancy rate per puncture and transfer, and lastly the number of children born from October 1982 through 1987. Follicular puncture was performed pelviscopically in 1982-1986. Since April 1986 vaginosonographically guided follicular puncture without anaesthesia has been used in more than 95% of the patients.

Out of the 67 patients enrolled in this study, who underwent down regulation before and/or along with HMG or FSH stimulation, only 55 patients proceeded to follicular puncture. Table 2 shows the individual causes of drop out in the cancelled cycles, where further stimulations were stopped between the 4th and 14th day of the cycle.

In group 1 the GnRH test, using 100µg i.v, was performed on the second cycle day and it was negative in all but 3 patients of this group. Therefore, further down regulation with 500µg decapeptyl daily was applied for 6 days in these cases till the test turned negative. HMG or FSH stimulation was carried out, taking into consideration the individual oestradiol responses of the patient (Tables 2 and 3).

Table 2. Dropout list. Decapeptyl-HMG-stimulation for IVF/ET.

Group	Patients	Follicular Punctures	Not Punctured Patients	Comments
I	27	21	6	
			1	resistant sperm contamination by chlamydia
			2	
			3	unsufficient E_2-response compared to number of follicles
			4	
			5	
			6	
II	40	34	6	
			1	ovarian cyst formation (>6 cm)
			2	
			3	unsufficient E_2-response compared to number of follicles
			4	
			5	
			6	

Table 3. Decapeptyl-, HMG-, HCG-Stimulation. IVF/ET (1987).

Group	Patients	Follicular Puncture		Oocytes Per Puncture		Transfers		Embryos Per Transfer	Pregnancies	Per FP	Per ET
	n	n	%	n	$\bar{x}$	n	%	$\bar{x}$	n	%	%
1	27	21	78	157	7	15	73	3	6	27	38
2	40	34	85	221	6	27	79	3	6	17	21
Total	67	55	82	378	6.5	42	76	3	12	22	30

Follicular puncture was performed in 78% and 85% of the patients in group 1 and 2, respectively. All of the recovered oocytes, about 6-7 oocytes/patient, were incubated with the husband's sperms. Embryotransfer was carried out in 73% and 79% of the cases subjected to follicular puncture in groups 1 and 2, respectively. The pregnancy rate per follicular puncture and per embryo transfer are shown in detail in Table 3.

DISCUSSION

Our sixty-seven patients who received decapeptyl, in spite of simultaneous gonadotropic stimulation, were not a favorable group to demonstrate the success of IVF/ET. These patients had premature LH surges during previous stimulation cycles and insufficient follicular development. LH rises could be suppressed in all patients with the GnRH analogue. The mode of application of this GnRH agonist influenced the stimulation with HMG, as higher doses of HMG were necessary to achieve optimal follicular maturation. In 12 cases, 6 in each group, follicular puncture was not performed due to a deficient oestradiol response following down-regulation and gonadotropic stimulation. In the absence of an appropriate increase in follicular size and maturity, follicular punctures are not justified. We consider that allthough vaginosonographically guided operative interventions are easy they should be performed only when there is a reasonable chance to achieve pregnancy after IVF and ET. In one case, chlamydial infection of the husband's sperms was detected only after the start of stimulation; and in another case in group 2, a big ovarian cyst developed around day 6. It was punctured vaginosonographically, but the patient preferred to stop further stimulation in this cycle.

The onset of application of GnRH analogue and the start of gonadotropic stimulation is of great significance. In three patients in group 1, down-regulation was performed over 3 weeks, as the GnRH test showed persistent FSH/LH releases.

The action of GnRH analogues at the level of the adenohypophysis inhibits gonadal function through suppression of the gonadotropins. Yet, a direct action at the gonadal level can not be excluded. GnRH analogues allow a better control of the ovarian function and application of gonadotropins. Further comparative studies with evaluation of the achieved pregnancies are needed to decide whether down-regulation should be applied at the start [8] or in the middle of the cycle by daily pulses or with a depot slow releasing capsule. Also, it remains to be seen if it is better to continue Decapeptyl administration until the occurrence of pregnancy or to stop on the day of HCG administration.

Indications for applying decapeptyl in induction of ovulation with simultaneous or subsequent administration of gonadotropins are:

1. Premature LH surges in previous cycles.
2. Previous overstimulation reaction of the ovaries after HMG stimulation.
3. Polycystic ovaries.
4. Hyperandrogenic ovarian insufficiency.
5. Resistant ovary syndrome.

We suggest also that decapeptyl should be used not only in patients with premature LH rises and other pathological ovarian reactions, but also in patients with normal cycles in order to achieve a more homogenous state of follicular development.

REFERENCES

1. Mettler, L, Michelmann, HW, Riedel, H-H, Grillo, M, Weisner, D and Semm, K (1984). In-vitro-fertilization and embryo replacement at the Department of Obstetrics and Gynecology, University of Kiel, FRG, IVF 4, 250

2. Williams, RF and Hodgen, GD, (1980). Disparate effects of human chorionic gonadotrophin during the late follicular phase in monkeys: normal ovulation, follicular atresia, ovarian acyclicity, and hypersecretion of follicle-stumulating hormone. Fertil Steril, 33, 61

3. Trounson, AQ (1983). Factors controlling normal embryo development and implantation of human oocytes fertilized in vitro. In: Beier, HM and Lindner, HR (eds.) "Fertilization of the Human Egg in Vitro". p.235. (Springer: Berlin)

4. Belchetz, PE, Plant TM, Nakai, Y, Koegh, EJ and Knobil, E (1978). Hypophysial responses to continuous, and intermittent delivery of hypothalamic gonadotrophin-releasing hormone. Science, 202, 631

5. Wild, L, Häusler, A, Hutchison, JS, Marschall, O and Knobil, E (1981). Estradiol as a gonadotrophin releasing hormone in the rhesus monkey. Endocrinology, 108, 2011

6. Coy, DH, Vilchez-Martinez, JA, Coy, EJ and Schally, AV (1976). Analogues of luteinizing hormone releasing hormone with increased biological activity produced by D-amino acid. J Med Chem, 19, 423

7. Michelmann, HW, Tinneberg, H-R, Weisner, D, and Mettler, L, (1987). Follikelpunktion im Rahmen der menschlichen in-vitro-Fertilization. Geburtsh u Frauenheik, 47, 598
8. Wildt, L, Diedrich, K, V D Ven, H, Al Hasani, S, Hübner, H and Klasen, R(1986). Ovarian hyperstimulation for in-vitro fertilization controlled by GnRH agonist administered in combination with human menopausal gonadotrophins. Human Reprod, 1, 15

15

INDUCTION OF OVULATION WITH THE COMBINATION OF LHRH ANALOG IN A SHORT PROTOCOL AND EXOGENOUS GONADOTROPINS

P. BARRIERE, P. LOPES and **B. CHARBONNEL**
IVF Department, CHU Nantes
44035 - Nantes Cedex 01, France

INTRODUCTION

A better control of ovarian hyperstimulation is an important element in improving results of in vitro fertilization (IVF). Many existing therapeutic protocols utilise substances like clomiphene citrate (CC), human gonadotropins (HMG) or GnRH. Because of the overall satisfactory results, the gonadotropins alone or associated with clomiphene citrate have generally been used in the induction of ovulation. However, there are two major drawbacks in these regimens. A proportion of patients show a poor reproductive response due to poor follicular development. The presence of frequent spontaneous LH surges and even elevated LH levels during the late follicular phase before the induction of ovulation by HCG influences the results. To avoid these endogenous pituitary interferences, the production of reversible medical hypophysectomy, by use of GnRH analogs, has been advocated.

Buserelin (Suprefact-Hoechst) has been reported to suppress endogenous LH surges and to improve HMG-induced multifollicular ovulation for IVF. The GnRH analog was usually started 2 to 3 weeks prior to gonadotropins, in order to obtain pituitary desensitization [1]. As reported by Fleming et al., [2], we have used a short protocol starting from the second day of the cycle, employing both the gonadotropins and [D-Trp^6]GnRH (IPSEN-BIOTECH, Paris) in order to exploit the initial flare-up effect and the succeeding blockade of the hypophysis. In a preliminary, prospective and randomised study, we have shown a significant rise in the pregnancy rate per induction cycle as compared with a CC-HMG protocol [3]. We present here the follow up of this study as compared with CC-HMG in 122 cycles. In relation to the better results in the pregnancy rate per cycle, this short analog-HMG regimen has become our regular first choice protocol.

PATIENTS METHODS

Indications for IVF were: blocked tubes, idiopathic infertility of over 4 years, failure of artificial insemination with donor sperm, male factor, endometriosis and dysovulation refractory to conventional therapeutic measures.

STUDY DESIGN

The patients were divided into 2 groups. Group I contained 59 patients in whom 79 cycles were induced with [D-Trp^6]GnRH-HMG. Group II represented 42 patients in whom 43 cycles were induced with CC-HMG. Group III was composed of 25 patients who failed CC-HMG and were renetered into GnRH analog treatment.

For group I the treatment consisted of daily subcutaneous injection of [D-Trp^6]GnRH (100µg from day 2 until induction by HCG) and HMG 75 to 300 IU/day, doses being adjusted in relation to the ovarian response. The induction of ovulation by 10000 IU of HCG, was effected according the usual criteria of follicular maturation (relationship between estradiol level and number of follicles exceeding 14mm in diameter).

In group II treatment consisted of 100mg of CC daily from day 2 to day 6 of HMG (75 to 225 IU per day from day 2 in doses adjusted for ovarian response).

The ovarian response was monitored by daily estimation of estradiol levels from the second day and 3 or 4 ultrasonographic ovarian scannings. The oocyte retrieval was effected 34 hours after the HCG injection by means of laparoscopies in 64% of cases and was ultrasound guided in 36%. In all cases, the luteal phase was maintained by HCG, if the estradiol level was less than 1500pg/ml on the induction day or micronised oral progesterone, if it was otherwise.

There were no significant differences in the clinical features of patients between the 2 groups, with respect to age (32.8±3.5 years vs 33.2±3.8 years) and various causes of infertility. Statistical analysis was done with chi-square test.

GROUP RESULTS

In group I, there was a significant reduction in the number of cancellations before oocyte recovery as compared with group II. This may have been partially due to the total absence of premature LH surges in group I (Table 1).

There was a significant rise in the estradiol level and the number of large follicles, in group I as compared with group II.

Table 1. Cancellations before oocyte recovery.

Reason for Cancellation	Group I	Group II	P
Low estradiol	4	4	
Estradiol decrease	1	0	
Cysts >25 mm	2	0	
LH surge	0	11	p<0.01
TOTAL	7/79	15/43	p<0.01

However the correlation between the estradiol level and the number of large follicles remained the same in both groups.

There was also a significant rise in the number of recovered mature oocytes and cleaved embryos in group I. This increase in the number of embryos resulted in a significant rise in number of patients who could benefit from cryopreservation of embryos (Table 2).

Table 2. Folliculogenesis comparisons.

Parameter Used	Group I	Group II	P
Estradiol on HCG day	1920 ± 1058	1471 ± 617	<0.05
Large follicles	6.26 ± 2.97	4.86 ± 1.92	<0.05
E_2/large follicle	306	302	
Mature oocytes	4.1 ± 2.71	2.26 ± 2.01	<0.01
Cleaved embryos	2.9 ± 2.21	1.64 ± 1.59	<0.01

The pregnancy rate remained the same when related to embryo transfer, whereas it was considerably increased in relation to oocyte retrieval. The pregnancy rate per induction cycle was significantly increased in group I (Table 3). There was no difference in the spontaneous abortion rate between the two groups (5 of 25 versus 1 of 6).

Table 3. Pregnancy rate comparisons.

Parameter Used	Group I	Group II	P
Per induction cycle	31.6%	13.9%	<0.05
Per oocyte recovery	34.7%	21.4%	
Per embryo transfer	36.8%	31.6%	

Analysis of the results for the 25 patients in group III demonstrates the advantages of this method over CC-HMG.

When these patients were treated with the group I protocol there was a significant decrease in the number of cancellations before oocyte recovery (12 of 26 with CC due in 8 to LH surges and in 4 to low responses), as compared with 2 out of 29 in group III (2 low responses). The number of mature oocytes and cleaved embryos was significantly increased with the group III protocol (Table 4).

Table 4. Results in patients transferring from group II to group III protocol.

13 Patients	Group II Protocol (14 oocytes recovered)	Group III Protocol (12 oocytes recovered)	P
Estradiol	1416 ± 623	1940 ± 804	
Large follicles	4.78 ± 1.93	6.06 ± 2.35	
Mature oocytes	1.5 ± 1.45	3.67 ± 2.27	<0.01
Cleaved embryos	1.0 ± 1.1	2.92 ± 2.15	<0.01
Pregnancy	0	4	

Sixty three pregnancies defined by elevation of ß HCG and visualisation of a gestational sac on the ultrasound scanning were obtained after 297 inductions. The breakdown of these pregnancies by presenting indication is shown in Table 5.

There was no change in the initial pregnancy rate with respect to the age of the patient. However the number of spontaneous abortions was increased after 35 years (Table 6).

The relationship between the pregnancy rate and the dose of HMG shows a fall in the pregnancy rate with a rise in the dose of

Table 5. Pregnancy rates by presenting etiology.

Etiology	Percent of Study Population	Pregnancy Rate
Tubal	64.6%	21.1%
Idiopathic and AID failure	20.9%	36.5%
Endometriosis	9.2%	30.4%
Dysovulation	1.7%	25.0%
Male factor	3.6%	22.2%

HMG (Table 7). Significantly larger amounts of HMG had been used in cycles that were not followed by pregnancy.

Table 6. Pregnancy rate breakdown by age of patient.

Age	Initial Pregnancy Rate (Third Trimester Rate)
$\leq$ 30 years	25.5% (22.2%)
30 < age $\leq$ 35 years	24.4% (19.5%)
> 35 years	27.8% (13.9%)

This was independent of the duration of stimulation and body weight of the patient.

Table 7. Relationship between HMG dose and pregnancy rate.

HMG Doses/Induction	Initial Pregnancy Rate (Third Trimester Rate)
$\leq$ 10 vials	40.0% (28.0%)
10 < vials $\leq$ 25	26.7% (20.9%)
> 25 vials	13.5% (11.5%)

The initial pregnancy rate was satisfactory when the estradiol level exceeded 2500pg/ml on the HCG day. However, there was then an increased number of spontaneous abortions (32%).

Because of the poor predictive value of the estradiol level on HCG day, we studied the kinetics of the estradiol level on the days preceding the HCG injection. We found that the cycles that are associated with pregnancy show significantly increased estradiol levels on days 4, 5 and 6 before HCG administration. This enabled us to determine favourable conditions for pregnancy, in relation to duration of estradiol rise (Table 8).

Table 8. Correlation between duration of E_2 rise prior to HCG and pregnancy rate.

Duration of E_2 Rise	Cycles	Initial Pregnancy Rate (Third Trimester Rate)
Non-analysable	21	9.5% (9.5%)
4 days	29	10.3% (0%)
5 days	82	13.4% (12.2%)
6 days	88	36.3% (28.3%)
7 days	29	51.7% (41.4%)

DISCUSSION

The use of [D-Trp^6]GnRH in association with gonadotropins, from the second day, has improved the results of in vitro fertilization when compared with the usual protocols. Use of a GnRH analog completely suppresses the spontaneous LH surges and premature luteinization of follicles. It has been shown that spontaneous LH surges significantly reduce the pregnancy rate [4, 5, 6]. In addition the monitoring of weak spontaneous surges besides the usual LH surges, as described by Wolf and al [7], is difficult.

An elevated LH level during the follicular phase is associated with poor results in vitro fertilization [8]. Recently Ben Rafael [9] showed that the rate of polyspermia is more frequent in the oocytes derived from luteinized follicles (determined by a rise in progesterone in the follicular fluid).

The biological activity of LH can be modified by GnRH analogs. Meldrum [10] had shown during treatment with a GnRH analog that the biological activity of LH is diminished. This observation becomes much more significant, if we consider Abuzeid [11] who suggests that the endogenous or exogenous LH could show a relatively elevated bioactivity particularly in the presence of elevated estradiol levels.

GNRH analogs enable us to lower basal LH, suppress premature luteinization and LH surges, and obtain better timing of induction with HCG, without the fear of endogenous interference. These benefits, that are obtained after a prolonged desensitization, are also obtained with the short protocol.

The improvement in folliculogenesis could be explained by the following hypothesis: The flare up effect (initial release of endogenous LH and FSH), observed from day 2 to day 3 could play a role in the recruitment of follicles. However such an improvement is also obtained after desensitization in a long administration protocol [12].

The influence of GnRH and its agonists on the ovary is now proved from several studies in animals. Eppig [13] has shown an action on the granulosa cells of the follicles in rats; he noted the influence of GnRH on the synthesis and liberation of arachidonic acid from the granulosa cells and an ability to induce meiotic maturation of oocytes. In humans, Bramley [14] has demonstrated specific binding sites for GnRH and its agonists in luteal homogenates. These observations raise the possibility that GnRH analogs could have a role in intragonadal regulation of human luteal function.

Improvement in folliculogenesis could also be linked to the use of increased quantity of HMG. However there was no positive correlation between HMG dose and pregnancy rate. On the contrary, our results showed a relative fall in the pregnancy rate with increased HMG. The increase in dose in the patients who do not conceive is independent of the body weight. Although it has been shown that the average dose of HMG increases with the weight, some patients presenting an hypoestrogenic state in fact require increased amounts of HMG, irrespective of their weight [15].

There is no negative effect of the analogs on the cleavage or implantation rates. There may even be an improvement in the quality of recovered oocytes or embryos, by prevention of premature luteinization. The rate of spontaneous abortions is not increased. No anomalies have been observed in 49 children born following this treatment. We do note an increase in the rate of spontaneous abortions with the rise in age of the patients and in cycles where the estradiol level exceeded 2500pg/ml on the day of HCG. This is in agreement with the observations of Salat-Baroux [16].

According to different teams, GnRH analogs could be used in a short protocol (stimulation by gonadotropins from the onset of agonist therapy) or a long protocol (stimulation by gonadotropins after the establishment of gonadotropin insufficiency by the agonist). Whatever has been the mode of administration of agonist, the different teams conclude there is an improvement in the recruitment of follicles with better results in terms of pregnancy. Porter [17] has observed that the results are almost identical with the 2 protocols in spite of the varying mode of administration of analogs. Zorn [18] also obtained similar results in terms of pregnancy when he compared 215 cycles in the long protocol and 141 cycles in the short protocol, although the study was not randomised.

Nevertheless we can identify situations that are more favourable to the use of one protocol or the other. For example, in the short protocol we can exploit the initial flare-up produced at the onset of GnRH analog administration. The dose of gonadotropins and that of the agonist is 2 or 3 times less . The cost of the cycle and the therapeutic duration are therefore reduced as compared with the long protocol. However, in the long protocol, the prior establishment of gonadotropic insufficiency enables us to fix the time of gonadotropin stimulation and to program the cycle.

It has been shown in the monkey that the initial level of gonadotropins is predictive of the rapidity of desensitization with GnRH antagonists [19]. It is conceivable that a sub-group of population could benefit from prolonged suppression of LH, consequently the long protocol could be better adapted to their clinical profiles.

The initial "flare-up" effect is more important with respect to LH than with FSH. Hence the possibility of development of functional cysts or the stimulation of cells, elaborating progesterone are in general avoided in the long protocol. However, this does not seem to be a frequent drawback in the short protocol (3% in our series).

The repeated failure of induction in IVF has given rise to the concept of low responders which include different criteria according to the different teams. As per our criteria subjects who show premature endogenous LH surges are not included in this concept. Lyles has noted the low recurrence frequency of LH surges and cyst formation among women undergoing repeat cycles of ovulation induction for IVF, as opposed to recurrence of poor response [20]. We limit it to those cases of failures with defective folliculogenesis, in spite of well adapted dose of gonadotropins. Neveu [12] includes subjects who showed a negative response to clomiphene on at least 2 occasions, adding also the existence of premature LH surges. A study of 50 cycles in her criteria showed an oocyte recovery rate of 70% and a pregnancy rate of 20% when treated with GNRH analogs. Belaish [21] defines her group of low responders as those who showed premature LH surges, insufficient and low estradiol levels and recovery of one ococyte or absence of oocyte. Under buserelin-FSH-HMG, a pregnancy rate of 23,5% per cycle is obtained. She further showed that better results with agonists are realised in patients who showed premature LH surges in the previous cycles.

However, the problem of poor responses is not completely solved by analogs. Kenigsberg [22] after having utilised GnRH antagonist in low responder monkeys had suggested that poor response may be related to ovarian causes. Neveu [23] also shares this view. She raises the possibility of the existence of endogenous pathology related to adhesions being responsible for the poor development of follicles.

The decision to inject HCG is often arbitrary [24], but with the analogs, the timing of HCG administration is not critical. However, the optimal timing of HCG injection should be based not only on the level of estrogen but also on the duration of estradiol rise.

The kinetics of estradiol levels on the HCG day as well as the day prior to and after HCG, are often more predictive of the outcome of the cycle in IVF, than the absolute value attained. Our data show that certain kinetics of stimlation yield better results, based on the estradiol rise for at least 6 days prior to induction. This notion of duration of estradiol kinetics has already been reported in usual protocols with slight variations in the modalities but the optimal period of six days was stressed [25, 26, 27]. Sarutskie and al [28] in the evaluation of preovulatory hormone profiles showed that every protocol is linked to a certain hormone profile, that gives an optimal number of good quality oocytes and optimal quality of luteal phase.

This study shows the benefits obtained in IVF by using [D-Trp^{6}]GnRH in a short protocol. This enables us to obtain optimal conditions for ovarian stimulation: optimal use of the analog, low dose of HMG and adapting its dose to obtain an estrogen rise for 6 or 7 days. If this profile is not achieved it is preferable not to go ahead with induction.

REFERENCES

1. Porter, RN, Smith, W, Caret, IL, Abdul Wahid, NA and Jacobs, HS (1984). Induction of ovulation for in vitro fertilisation using Buserelin and gonadotropins. Lancet, ii, 1284

2. Fleming, R, Haxton, MJ, Yates, RWS, Conaghan, C and Coutts, JRT (1985). A simple procedure for the induction of multiple follicular growth with blockage of the LH surge in normal women. Program of 67th Annual Meeting of the Endocrine Society, Baltimore, Maryland, USA, Abstract, 149

3. Barriere, P, Lopes, P, Boiffard, JP, Pousset, C, Quentin, M, Sagot, P, L'Hermite, A, Lerat, MF and Charbonnel, B (1987). Use of GNRH analogues in ovulation induction for IVF: benefit of a short administration regimen. J IVF-ET, 4, 64

4. Eibschitz, I, Belaisch-Allart, J and Frydman, R (1986). In vitro fertilization management and results in stimulated cycles with spontaneous LH discharge. Fertil Steril, 45, 231

5. Nader, S, Berkowitz, AS, Maklad, N, Wolf, DP and Held, B (1986). Characteristics of patients with and without gonadotropin surges during follicular recruitement in an in vitro fertilization embryo transfer program. Fertil Steril, 45, 75

6. Lejeune, B, Degueldre, M, Camus, M, Vekemans, M, Opsomer, L and Leroy, F (1986). In vitro fertilisation and embryo transfer as related to endogenous LH rise or HCG administration. Fertil Steril, 45, 377

7. Wolf, P, Ochs, D, Nader, S and Berkowitz, A (1986). Undetected ovulation in in vitro fertilization - embryo transfer patients. Fertil Steril, 5, 892

8. Howles, CM, Mc Namee, MC, Edwards, RG, Goswamy, R and Steptoe, PC (1986). Effect of high tonic levels of luteinizing hormone on outcome in vitro fertilization. Lancet, ii, 521
9. Ben Rafael, Z, Meloni, F, Strauss, JF, Blasco, L, Mastroianni, L and Flickinger, GL (1987). Relationships between polypronuclear fertilization and follicular fluid hormones in gonadotropin treated women. Fertil Steril, 47, 284
10. Meldrum, DR, Tsad, Z, Monroe, SE, Braunstein, GD, Sladek, J, Vale, W, Lu, JKH, Rivier, J, Judd, HL and Chang, RJ (1984), Stimulation of LH fragments with reduced bioactivity following GNRH agonist administration in women. J Clin Endocrin Metab, 58, 755
11. Abuzeid, MI and Yeoman, R (1987). Luteinizing hormone bioactivity in human menopausal gonadotropin, human chorionic gonadotropin - induced cycles. Fertil Steril, 47, 238
12. Neveu, S, Hedon, B, Bringer, J, Chincholle, JM, Arnal, F, Humeau, C, Cristol, P and Viala, JL (1987). Ovarian stimulation by a combination of a GNRH agonist and gonadotropins in IVF. Fertil Steril, 47, 639
13. Eppig, JJ (1986). Action de la LHRH sur l'ovaire. Contracept Fertil Sexualte, 14, 859
14. Bramley, TA, Menzies, GS and Baird, DT (1985). Specific binding of gonadotrophin-releasing hormone and an agonist to human corpus luteum homogenates: characterization, properties and luteal phase levels. J Clin Endocrinol Metab, 61, 834
15. Chong, AP, Rafael, RW and Forte, CC (1986). Influence of weight in the induction of ovulation with HMG and HCG. Fertil Steril, 46, 599
16. Salat-Baroux, J, Cornet, D, Antoine, JM, Alvarez, S, Alfiere, L and Bonnardot, JP (1987). Un cas de stimulation grave au cours d'une fecondation in vitro suivie de grossesse. Gynecologie, 38, 113
17. Porter, R, Smith, W, Craft, I, Abdul Wahid, N and Jacobs, H (1986). Induction of multifollicular development for IVF using buserelin and gonadotropins: clinical and endocrine results. J IVF-ET, 3, 174
18. Zorn, JR(1987). Les analogues de la LHRH et les nouvelles techniques d'induction de l'ovulation pour la fecondation in vitro et le transfert intratubaire des gametes. Contracept Fertil Sexualte, 15, 771
19. Chillick, CF, Itskovitz, J, Hahn, DW, McGuire, JL, Danforth, DR and Hodgen GD (1987). Characterizing pituitary response to the gonadotropin releasing hormone antagonist in monkeys: tonic follicle stimulating hormone/luteinizing hormone secretion versus acute GnRH challenge tests before, during and after treatment. Fertil Steril, 48, 480
20. Lyles, R, Gibbons, WE, Dodson, MG, Poindexter, AN, Young, RL, Rossavik, IK and Findley, WE (1985). Characterization and response of women undergoing repeat cycles of ovulation induction in an in vitro fertilization and embryo transfer program. Fertil Steril, 44, 832

21. Belaish-Allart, J, Frydman, R, Fries, N and Testart, J (1986). FSH purifiee et fecondation in vitro. Contracept Fertil Sexualte, 14, 697
22. Kenigsberg, D, Littman, BA, Williams, R and Hodgen, GD (1984). Medical hypophysectomy - Variability of ovarian response to gonadotrophin therapy. Fertil Steril, 42, 116
23. Neveu, S, Hodon, B, Mares, P, Bringer, J, Arnal, F, Deschamps, F, Cristol, P and Humeau, P (1987). Experience en FIV d'un agoniste du GNRH: la Buserelin. Contr Fertil Sexualte, 14, 774
24. Messinis, TE and Templeton, A (1986). Urinary oestrogen levels and follicle ultrasound measurement in clomifene induced cycles with an endogenous LH surge. Brit J Obstet Gynecol, 93, 43
25. Friedrich, W, Lire, K, Korner, H and Wilken, T (1986). The follicular phase stimulated by human pituitary gonadotrophin and the luteal phase following IVF. Exptl Clin Endocrinol, 87, 1
26. Levran, D, Lopata, A, Nayerden, PL, Martin, MJ, McBain, JC, Baylay, CM, Speirs, AL and Johnston, WIH (1985). Analysis of the outcome of IVF in relation to the timing of HCG administration by the duration of estradiol rise in stimulated cycles. Fertil Steril, 44, 335
27. Quigley, MM, Sokoloski, JE and Richards, SI (1985). Timing HCG administration by days of oestradiol rise. Fertil Steril, 44, 791
28. Zarutskie, PW, Kuzan FB, Dixon, L, Soules, MR (1987). Endocrine changes in the late follicular and postovulatory intervals as determinants of the IVF pregnancy rate. Fertil Steril, 47, 137

16

THE USE OF GnRH ANALOGUES FOR SYNCHRONIZATION OF OOCYTE DONATION

P. DEVROEY, M. CAMUS, J. De SCHACHT, I. KHAN, J. SMITZ, C. STAESSEN, L. Van WAESBERGHE, A. WISANTO and A.C. Van STEIRTEGHEM
Centre for Reproductive Medicine, Medical Campus,
Vrije Universiteit Brussel, Laarbeeklaan 101, 1090 Brussels, Belgium

INTRODUCTION

Since the first pregnancy and delivery in a patient with absent ovaries [1] more pregnancies have been reported after oocyte donation. Synchrony of the donor's and recipient's cycles is mandatory. We here report the synchronization of the donor's cycle to the recipient's substituted cycle using a long and short protocol of GnRH analogues in combination with hMG and HCG.

MATERIALS AND METHODS

From June 1, 1987 until December 1, 1987 GnRH analogues have been to synchronize the donor's and recipient's cycles in our oocyte donation programme. Ten patients agreed to donate their oocytes, 3 patients had a concomitant tubal ligation and seven were volunteers. Four donors were known and six were anonymous. The mean age of the donors was 28.9 years (range 25-34 years).

Twenty-one recipients were accepted. Twenty women suffered from primary ovarian failure and one patient with functional ovaries was included because she had a chromosomal translocation (46,XX,t(pt;12)(p11;11).

The mean age of the recipients was 32 years (range 23-41 years). In 8 donors [D-Ser(tBu)^6,Pro^{9}NHEt]LHRH, buserelin, was administered intranasally 6 times daily in a long protocol that started on day 21 of the natural cycle. HMG was started on the day corresponding to the first day of the recipient's cycle.

In two donor patients 100µg buserelin was given intranasally 6 times daily from the first day of the menstrual period in association with hMG (short protocol of buserelin administration).

The administration of hMG was adapted in the short and the long protocol as earlier described [2]. HCG was injected when serum 17ß-oestradiol (E2) was at least 1500ng/l in the presence of 6 follicles with a diameter of at least 18mm.

Buserelin treatment was continued during the luteal phase until the onset of the next menstrual bleeding. Oocyte retrieval was done 36 hours after hCG by laparoscopy in 5 patients and under ultrasound guidance in another 5 [3]. Donated oocytes were inseminated with sperm of the recipient's husband and replaced as fertilized oocytes (n=60 [4] or as 4-cell embryos (n=15) [5]).

The remaining embryos were cryopreserved for later use [6-9]. The 20 patients without ovarian function were treated with oestradiol valerate (days 1-5: 1mg, days 6-9: 4mg, days 10-13: 6mg, days 14-17: 2mg, days 18-26: 4mg, days 27-28: 1mg). Progesterone was injected 50mg intramuscularly on day 14: and 100mg from days 15 to 26 [10]. In 15 out of 20 recipients with primary ovarian failure, the scheme had to be adapted in relation to the unpredictable length of the donor's follicular phase. In the patient with functional ovaries the embryos were replaced in a natural cycle. The donation programme was approved by the Ethical Committee of the hospital [11].

RESULTS

In the 8 patients with the long protocol the mean duration of desensitization prior to hMG administration was 19 days (range: 12-33). The mean length of the follicular phase was 12 days (range: 10-13).

In the two donors with the short protocol, the length of the follicular phase was 11 and 15 days respectively . The mean

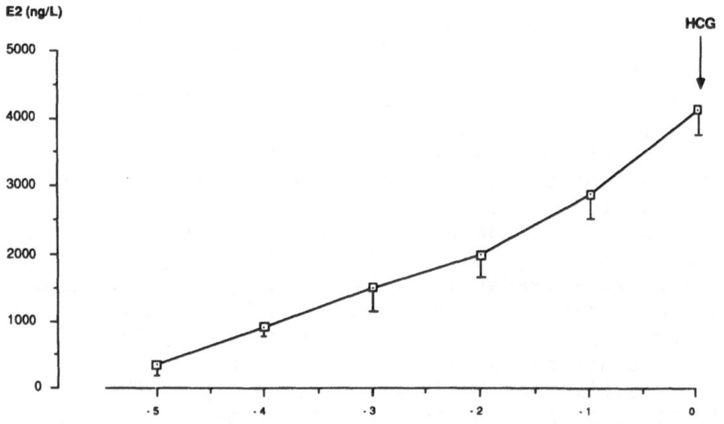

FIGURE 1 The mean concentration of 17ß-oestradiol (E_2ng/l) after the combined stimulation with buserelin and human menopausal gonadotrophins on days hCG -5, -4, -3, -2, -1, and 0 in 10 donor patients

concentration of 17β-estradiol at the time of hCG administration was 4205ng/l (Fig. 1).

One hundred and fifty-eight oocytes were retrieved (mean 15.8; range 9-23) and 33 four-cell embryos were replaced in 15 uterine placements. Four pregnancies were established. Fifteen fertilized oocytes were replaced in 6 tubal placements. Two pregnancies were established (Table 1). The pregnancy rate was 28% per replacement and 11% per replaced embryo.

Table 1. Outcome of zygote or embryo transfers.

Site of placement	Transfers (n)	Embryos/ Zygotes (n)	Pregnancies (n)
Uterine	15	33	4
Fallopian tube	6	15	2
Total	21	48	6

The number of oocytes retrieved in known and anonymous donors, as well as the number of zygotes or embryos formed after insemination and the number of pregnancies are summarized in Table 2.

Table 2. Number of oocytes, embryos and pregnancies in known and anonymous oocyte donation.

Donors	Recipients	Oocytes	Zygote/Embryos		Pregnancies
			Fresh	Frozen	
Known (7)	8	116	23	36	2
Anonymous (3)	13	42	25	-	4
Total (10)	21	158	48	36	6

DISCUSSION

The synchronization of the cycles of donor and recipient patients is mandatory in an oocyte donation program. The administration of the GnRH analogue, buserelin, in the donor patient helps to fulfill this requirement.

If the long protocol of GnRH desensitisation is used, the hMG stimulation will be started in the donor patient on the first day of the artificial cycle of the acceptor. The duration of buserelin administration prior to the start of hMG can be adapted accordingly. Once the hMG is started the usual criteria of ovarian stimulation are used i.e. the dose of hMG will be dependent on the serum E_2 increase and the ultrasound findings; furthermore hCG will be administered when the usual criteria are met. It is impossible to predict the day of hCG administration in an individual patient. This individual variation can be solved by varying the day progesterone is started in the recipient. If hCG is given on day 14, no changes have to be made in the artificial cycle of the recipient. On the contrary when hCG is administered earlier or later, the start of oestradiol and progesterone administration will be advanced or retarded. In 8 donors receiving this long buserelin protocol only 4 patients received hCG on day 13, the remaining 4 donors had to receive hCG on day 12 (n=1), day 11 (n=2) or day 10 (n=1); the artificial cycles of the recipients were adapted accordingly.

Using the long GnRH protocol one can synchronize the cycles of donor and recipient by varying the start of hMG association in the donor, or by adapting the start of progesterone administration in the recipient depending on the moment of hCG administration in the donor.

For convenient reasons it can be indicated to use a short GnRH analogue protocol in the donor. Buserelin and hMG will be started on the first day of the menstrual period of the donor. In the recipient the low dose of oestradiol valerate will be continued until the stimulation can start in the donor. This means that the number of days that the recipient receives oestradiol valerate will vary according to the start of the buserelin-hMG association in the donor. As for the long protocol the day of hCG administration in the donor will again determine when progesterone and oestradiol will be started in the recipient. In donor VM hCG was given on day 11 and progesterone was started in the recipient on day 12. Donor VK started the buserelin-bMG combination after 3 years of oral contraception. The ovarian stimulation lasted 15 days. The 6 recipients continued to take 2mg oestradiol valerate until day 15, and the first dose of progesterone was given on day 16. The embryos were transferred on day 19; two out of six patients conceived.

In only 4 out of 10 cycles in the donor, the hCG was administered on day 13. In 16 recipients the first day of progesterone had to be advanced or delayed without compromising the establishment of pregnancies since 4 of these 16 recipients conceived.

The combination of GnRH analogue and hMG avoids the premature or endogenous LH surges. In this group of donor patients the mean number of retrieved oocytes (15.8) was about twice the mean number of eggs of our IVF-GIFT protocol. The corresponding mean serum oestradiol concentration at the time of hCG administration was also higher (4205ng/l). Since the oocytes were donated we did not have to consider the possible detrimental effect of the high oestrogen concentrations on the endometrium. The risk of an hyperstimulation syndrome was also reduced since we continued to administer buserelin until the onset of the next menstrual bleeding. Furthermore as reported earlier, the administration of GnRH analogues induces a luteal phase defect [12, 13].

The use of GnRH analogues in a donation program does not preclude the usefulness of an adequate freezing program [8, 9, 14]. In this study 36 embryos (42% of the total) were cryopreserved. Theoretically one can expect two more pregnancies when these frozen embryos are used. The high yield of oocytes and embryos in this protocol makes cryopreservation even more indicated.

For the 3 anonymous donations we accepted 13 recipients, who received a mean of 1.9 embryos. On the contrary the 7 known donations for 8 recipients yielded a mean of 7.3 embryos per recipient. For ethical reasons the number of embryos emplaced was limited to three and the remaining embryos were cryopreserved for later use. We obtained an acceptable pregnancy rate of 28% per transfer and an implantation rate of 11% per replaced embryo. More pregnancies might be expected when the cryopreserved embryos are transferred. This study indicates that the use of GnRH analogues in the donors allows for synchronization in a donation program.

ACKNOWLEDGEMENTS

We thank our nursing, technical and secretarial staff for their continuous support. A grant from the Belgian Fund for Medical Scientific Research is gratefully acknowledged.

REFERENCES

1. Lutjen, P, Trounson, A, Leeton, J, Findlay, J, Wood, C and Renou, P (1984). The establishment and maintenance of pregnancies using in vitro fertilization and embryo donation in a patient with primary ovarian failure. Nature, 307, 174

2. Devroey, P, Wisanto, A, Smitz, J, Braeckmans, P, Van Waesberghe, L and Van Steirteghem, AC (1987). Ovarian stimulation including in vitro fertilization. Ann Biol Clin, 45, 346

3. Wisanto, A, Braeckmans, P, Camus, M, Devroey, P. Khan, I, Staessen, C, Smitz, J, Van Waesberghe, L and Van Steirteghem, AC (1987). Perurethral ultrasound guided ovum pick-up. J Vitro Fertil Embryo Transfer, (in press)

4. Devroey, P, Braeckmans, P, Smitz, J, Van Waesberghe, L, Wisanto, A and Van Steirteghem, AC (1986). Pregnancy after translaparoscopic zygote intra-fallopian transfer in a patient with sperm antibodies. Lancet I, 1329.

5. Van Steirteghem, AC, Devroey, P, Heip, J, Liebaers, I, Liu, Y, Naaktgeboren, N, Olbrechts, H, Temmerman, M and Verhoeven, N (1984). Monitoring of patients in an in vitro fertilization and embryo transfer program. In: Bettocchi, S, Carenza, L, Loverro, G and Sadurny, G (eds.) "Human in Vitro Fertilization and Embryo Transfer and Early Embryo Development". p187 (Rome: CIC Edizioni Internationali)

6. Trounson, A and Mohr, L (1984). Human pregnancy following cryopreservation, thawing and transfer of an eight-cell embryo. Nature, 305, 707
7. Lasalle, B, Testart, J and Renard, JP (1985). Human embryo features that influence the success of cryopreservation with the use of 1, 2 propanediol. Fertil Steril, 44, 645
8. Van Steirteghem, AC, Van den Abbeel, E, Braechmans, P, Camus, M, Khan, I, Smitz, J, Staessen, C, Van Waesberghe, L, Wisanto, A and Devroey, P (1987). Pregnancy with a frozen-thawed embryo in a woman with primary ovarian failure. N Engl J Med, 317, 113
9. Van Steirteghem, AC, Van den Abbeel, E, Van Waesberghe, L, Braecknans, P, Khan, I, Nijs, M, Smitz, J, Staessen, C, Wisanto, A, and Devroey, P (1987). Cryopreservation of human embryos obtained after gamete intra-fallopian transfer and/or in vitro fertilization. Human Reprod, 2, 593
10. Navot, D, Laufer, N, Kopolovic, J, Rabinowitz, R, Birkenfeld, A, Lewin, A, Granat, Margalioth, EJ and Schenker, JG (1986). Artificially induced endometrial cycle and establishment of pregnancies in the absence of ovaries. N Engl J Med, 314, 806
11. Warnock, M (ed.) (1985). "A Question of Life". (Oxford: Basil Blackwell Ltd.)
12. Smitz, J, Devroey, P, Braeckmans, P, Camus, M, Khan, I. Staessen, C, Van Waesberghe, L, Wisanto, A and Van Steirteghem, AC (1987). Management of failed cycles in an IVF (GIFT) program with the combination of a GnRH analogue and hMG. Human Reprod, 2, 309
13. Devroey, P, Smitz, J, Camus, M, Deschacht, J, Van Waesberghe, L, Wisanto, A, Bourgain, Cl and Van Steirteghem, AC. La phase luteale apres traitement a la Busereline. Contrac Sexual Fertil (in press)
14. Devroey, P, Braeckmans, P, Camus, M, Khan, I, Smitz, J, Staessen, C, Van den Abbeel, E, Van Waesberghe, L, Wisanto, A and Van Steirteghem, AC (1987). Pregnancies after replacement of fresh and frozen-thawed embryos in a donation program. In: Feichtinger, N and Kemeter, P (eds.) "Future Aspects of Human In Vitro Fertilization" p.133. (Heidelberg: Springer-Verlag)

17

PROGRAMMED OOCYTE RETRIEVAL FOR IVF: CLINICAL AND BIOLOGICAL EFFECTS OF DIFFERENT PROTOCOLS OF PITUITARY SUPPRESSION AND FOLLICULAR STIMULATION

S. MASHIACH, Z. BEN-RAFAEL, A. ELENBOGEN, S. LIPITZ, J. BLANKSTEIN, D. LEVRAN, A. DAVIDSON, E. RUDAK and J. DOR
Interdepartmental Unit of Human Reproduction,
Department of Ob/Gyn, the Chaim Sheba Medical Center
and Sackler School of Medicine, Tel-Hashomer 52621, Israel

INTRODUCTION

The day of oocyte retrieval is the most important day in vitro fertilization (IVF) programs. It involves the coordination of the clinical, surgical and laboratory staff, thereby allowing only a limited number of cases to be performed daily. The day of retrieval depends on the day of menstruation and the individual ovarian response to medication, hence it is variable and can usually be anticipated only in the last few days of treatment. Some of these disadvantages can be overcome by fixing the day of retrieval in advance as in a "programmed cycle". Programmed IVF cycles include; suppression of the hypothalamic-pituitary-ovarian axis by oral contraceptives or gonadotropin releasing hormone (GnRH) analogues and a predetermined day for ovum pick-up. The method has been shown to be technically feasible and logistically desirable and can result in a clinical pregnancy rate equivalent to the more conventional individualized approaches to ovulation induction [1-6].

Programming of the cycle allows the use of the operating room to its full capacity without large fluctuations in the number of patients treated at any given day, the enrollment of patients into the program regardless of their day of menstruation [7] and it provides the staff and patients with a defined day for operation allowing time for planning and, thereby, reducing psychological stress.

We at the Sheba Medical Center have found it necessary to evaluate the diversities of ovarian responses following suppression of the hypothalamic-pituitary-ovarian axis by a GnRH analogue and to examine different protocols of follicular stimulation. In a series of studies we have examined protocols for pituitary suppression by GnRH analogue that varied in: (i) the length of suppression (15 days of suppression versus 30 days), (ii) the day of initiation of suppression (follicular or luteal phase) and (iii) the dose of GnRH analogue (daily administration versus controlled release (CR) preparation). We evaluated the effect of these variations on the length of the follicular phase, serum 17β estradiol (E_2) levels, the performance of oocytes in vitro and the pregnancy rate.

MATERIALS AND METHODS

Ninty two patients undergoing IVF and embryo transfer treatment were included in this study. The number of patients in each group is shown in Table 1. Only patients who were under 38 years of age,

Table I. Indications for cancellation before ovum pick-up.

	DECA 0.5 mg 15 Days +FSH/hMG	DECA 0.5 mg 30 Days +FSH/hMG	DECA 3.2 mg +FSH/hMG	DECA 3.2 mg +HMG (3 Amp.)	Control
No. of cases	20	21	20	15	16
Early luteinization	--	--	--	1 (6.6)	1 (6.2)
No response	1 (5)	3 (14.3)	2 (10)	--	--
Ovarian cysts	--	--	2 (10)	--	--
Total	1 (5)	3 (14.3)	4 (20)	1 (6.6)	1 (6.2)

with normal ovulatory cycles and infertility caused by tubal disease were selected. Ovum pick up was done via ultrasound.

We have prospectively studied two suppression protocols with GnRH analogue (Decapeptyl; Ferring). In the first, decapeptyl (0.5mg daily S.C.) was started on day 21 of the cycle (luteal phase), for either 15 or 30 days before ovarian stimulation was started and the same dose was continued during stimulation. In the second, decapeptyl Depot (3.2mg CR) was given as single injection on day 3 of the cycle (follicular phase). To assess the degree of suppression, a GnRH test was performed every week. This test indicated that the pituitary was completely suppressed one week after initiation of the analogue treatment.

These suppression protocols were followed by a stimulation protocol that was started either on day 16 (protocol 1 and 2) or on day 31 of suppression (protocol 1), with a fixed daily dose of 2 ampules/day of human menopausal gonadotropin (hMG; Teva Inc., Kefar Saba, Israel) supplemented with 2 ampules of pure follicle stimulating hormone (pure FSH; Teva, Israel) on days 1 and 2 only.

Since following suppression the "latent phase" is expected to be prolonged [6], we have examined whether this undesirable effect can be reversed by increasing the dose of hMG. Hence, we studied an additional group, where following suppression with Decapeptyl CR on day 3 of the cycle the patients were stimulated with an individualized high dose of hMG (3 ampules or more daily).

Follicular growth during gonadotropin treatment was assessed by daily measurements of serum E_2 levels and follicular size measured by ultrasonography (U/S), beginning on the first day of treatment. Human chorionic gonadotropin (hCG) was administered when E_2 reached levels above 400pg/ml and at least two follicles of 16mm diameter or more were observed in U/S at which time the daily injection of the analogue was discontinued. If no such response was achieved by day 15 of stimulation the cycle was cancelled. Daily plasma progesterone and luteinizing hormone (LH) levels to identify a premature LH surge or luteinization were also measured.

The control group consisted of patients that were not suppressed at all and stimulated with the same combination of hMG and pure FSH. Results are presented as mean ± standard error of the mean. Statistical analyses were performed using analysis of variance (Anova), Student's t-test, paired t-test and Chi Square where needed.

RESULTS

Serum E_2 levels on the day of hCG were similar in all the study groups. Evaluation of the trends in E_2 levels showed two distinct periods (Figure 1): A. the "latent phase" when E_2 levels are stationary and B. the "active phase" when E_2 levels

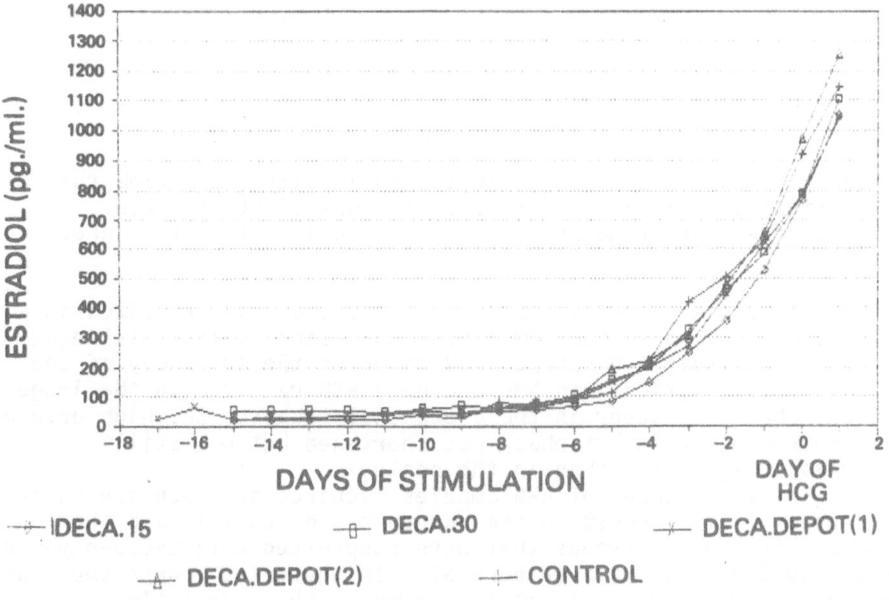

FIGURE 1 Mean serum E_2 levels, results are normalized to the day of hCG administration

are increasing daily. The first day of the active phase was considered as the day when the mean E_2 for the group increased significantly above the previous days levels. It was found that the mean number of days of the active phase was fairly constant around 6 to 7 days in all groups. Nevertheless, a large variation in the overall length of the follicular phase was noted between groups. Figure 2 displays the overall length of the follicular phase, from the first day of treatment to the day of hCG. Since the active phase was constant it is obvious that the large variation in the length of the follicular phase was due to variation in the latent phase.

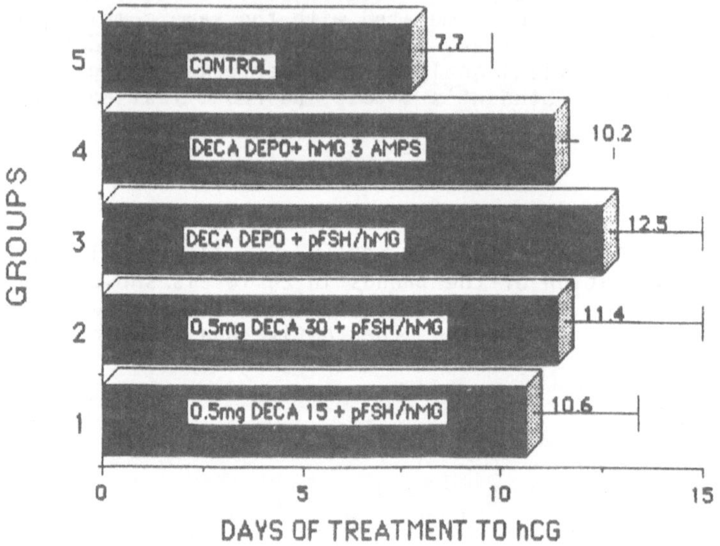

FIGURE 2 The overall length of the follicular phase from the first day of the treatment to the day of hCG in each suppression-stimulation protocol and in the control group

Fifteen days of suppression with 0.5mg daily resulted in a shorter latent phase than 30 days suppression, but still longer than the controls. Decapeptyl CR given on the third day of the cycle in combination with hMG and pure FSH resulted in the longest latent phase. However in the group that received the high dose of gonadotropin the latent phase was shortened but was still significantly longer than in the control.

The mean number of hMG ampules required to reach the desired response was the lowest in the unsuppressed controls and the highest in the two groups that were suppressed with Decapeptyl CR, from day 3 of the cycle (Figure 3). In these two groups the mean number of hMG ampules was equal, however, the stimulation period was shorter in the group that was treated with the higher daily dose of hMG

The number of oocytes recovered, a mean of about 6 to 7

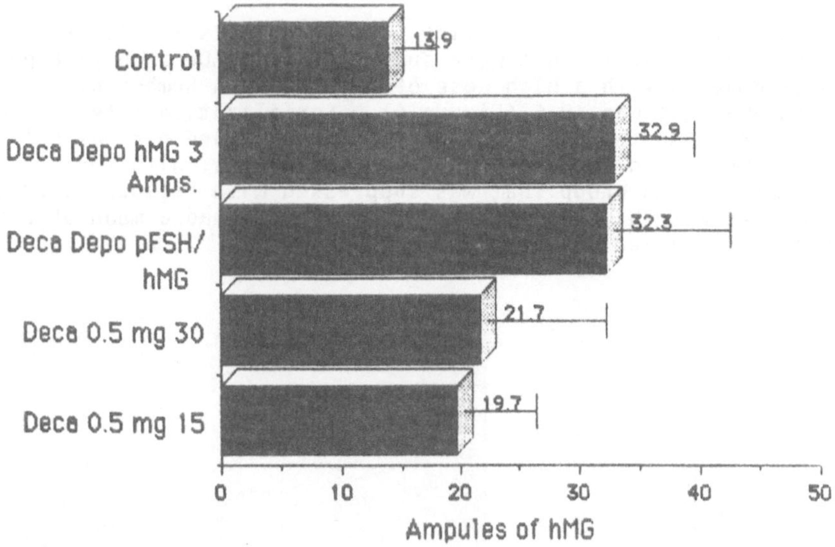

FIGURE 3 The mean number of hMG ampules used in each group

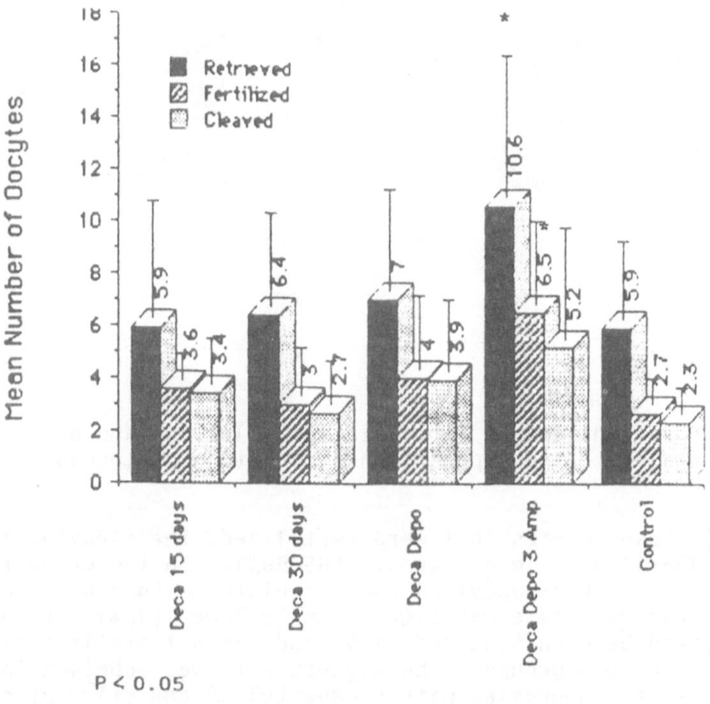

FIGURE 4 The number of oocytes recovered, fertilized and cleaved according to the suppression-stimulation protocols
*p<0.05 significantly higher than the other groups

oocytes per patient, was similar to the controls in all groups. However, in patients that were suppressed with Decapeptyl Depot and stimulated with a high dose of hMG the mean number of oocytes/patient was 10.6 (Figure 4). Fertilization rates (46%-61.4%) and the number of oocytes fertilizaed per patient (2.7-4) were also comparable between the groups, with the exception of the group that was suppressed with Decapeptyl CR and stimulated with high dose of hMG. This group had a mean of 6.5 oocytes fertilized (Figure 5).

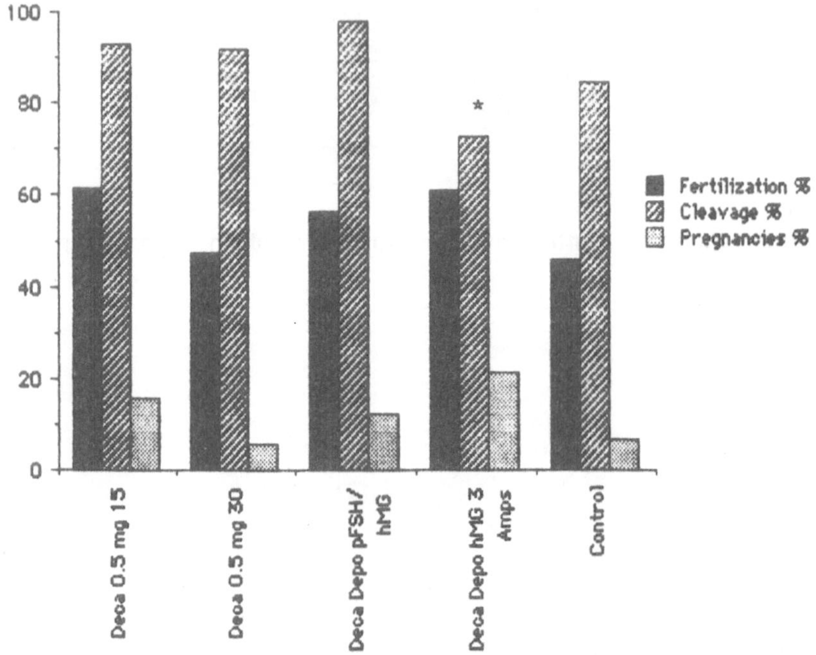

FIGURE 5 Percentages of fertilization, cleavage and pregnancies according to the suppression-stimulation protocols

Of those oocytes that were fertilized, the cleavage rates were similarly high in all groups (85-98%). In the group that was suppressed with Decapeptyl CR and stimulated with a high dose of hMG, the cleavage rate was significantly lower (73%). Pregnancy rates varied between 5.6% and 21.4% and was not statistically different between groups. The highest rate was acheived in the group that was suppressed with Decapeptyl CR and stimulated with the high dose of hMG. Cancellation rates varied between 5% to 20% and were not significantly different among the groups.

DISCUSSION

Frydman and colleagues and others [1-5] have successfully used a programmed cycle and a fixed day for hCG administration for oocyte retrieval without compromising the results compared to fully monitored control patients. The main purpose of this study was to investigate the impact of pituitary suppression by GnRH analogue on the length of the follicular phase, since the day of hCG administration and hence the feasibility of programming depends on the length of this period. We found that the latent part of the follicular phase was markedly prolonged with each protocol involving GnRH analogue compared to the control.

The day of hCG administration differs according to the duration of the suppression regimen, the dose, the phase of the cycle and the protocol for follicular maturation. We have therefore concluded that the follicular phase and the optimal day of hCG administration should be established prospectively for each suppression-stimulation protocol if programming is to be used.

The prolongation of the latent phase could be partially reversed by increasing the dose of hMG. Increasing the dose also resulted in a higher number of retrieved oocytes and a higher pregnancy rate. Although this study indicated that the day of hCG administration is highly variable and that a fixed day is difficult to establish thus preventing true programming, it seems that the use of the analogue (by virtue of preventing a premature LH surge) enables the postponement of hCG administration by one or two days thus avoiding the need to work on weekends.

The analogue prevents early luteinization which is the main cause for cancellation in routine IVF. Cancellation was not completely eliminated but this was due to inadequate response, despite continuous hMG administration for 15 days, or to cyst formation.

The prolongation of the latent phase in patients suppressed with the analogue indicates that the analogue induces ovarian hyposensitivity. This hyposensitivity can be reversed by

Table 2. Comparison between the results of IVF treatment following suppression with either Decapeptyl 0.5 or oral contraceptives for 15 days before stimulation.

	D-Trp^6-LHRH 0.5 mg 15 Days + FSH/hMG	Pill 15 Days + FSH/hMG
Days of stimulation	10.6 ± 2.63	10.6
Estradiol level on hCG day	766.5 ± 292	990 ± 218
No. of oocytes recovered	5.8 ± 4.5	6 ± 3.4
Fertilization rate (%)	61.4	62.9
Pregnancy rate/OPU (%)	15.7	34
Cancellation rate (%)	5	26

increasing the dose of hMG. Several theories can be offered to explain this observation [8-9] including suboptimal circulating levels of FSH due to pituitary down regulation; direct effect of the high dose of the analogue through low affinity binding sites to GnRH in the ovary; time required for a new cohort to grow due to possible disruption of folliculogenesis, and down regulation of FSH/LH receptors in the ovary caused by the 'flare-up' effect of the analogue.

In a previous study [6] we examined the feasibility of programming using oral contraceptives. We found that the best results were achieved when the oral contraceptives were given for the shortest period possible. Comparison of suppression with the oral contraceptives or GnRH analogue for 15 days (Table 2) shows that following oral contraceptive suppression the pregnancy rate was higher, however the cancellation rate was lower with the analogue.

In summary a GnRH analogue is an acceptable means to manipulate the cycle, however some unwarranted effects occur when GnRH analogue is given for extended periods or in high dose. Following prolonged suppression with GnRH analogue the latent phase which reflects a period of relative ovarian insensitivity is markedly prolonged. The ovarian desensitization that is encountered after the use of the analogue can be reversed by increasing the dose of hMG.

ACKNOWLEDGEMENT

We acknowledge Michal Kimhi for her excellent work in the laboratory.

REFERENCES

1. Templeton, A, Van Look, P, Lumsden, MA, Angell, R, Aitken, J, Duncan, AW and Baird, DT. (1984). The recovery of preovulatory oocytes using a fixed schedule of ovulation induction and follicle aspiration. Brit J Obstet Gynaecol, 91, 148

2. Braude, PR, Bright, MV, Douglas, CP, Milton, PJ, Robinson, RE, Williamson, JG, and Hutchinson, J (1984). A regimen for obtaining mature human oocytes from donors for research into human fertilization in vitro. Fertil Steril, 42, 34

3. Frydman, R, Forman, R, Rainhorn, JD, Belaisch-Allart, J, Hazout,A, amd Testart, J (1986) A new approach to follicular stimulation for in vitro fertilization: programmed oocyte retrieval. Fertil Steril, 46, 657

4. Frydman, R, Rainhorn, JD, Forman, R, Belaisch-Allart, J, Fernandez, H, Lassale, B and Testart, J (1986). Programmed oocyte retrieval during routine laparoscopy and embryo cryopreservation for later transfer. Am J Obstet Gynecol, 155, 112

5. Cohen, J, Debache, C, Solal, P, Serkine, AM, Achard, B, Boujenah, A, Pez, JP, Paris, X, Robert J, and Loffredo, V (1987). Results of planned in-vitro fertilization programming through the pre-administration of oestrogen-progesterone combined pill. Human Reproduction, 2, 7

6. Mashiach, S, Dor, J, Goldenberg, M, Shalev, J, Blankstein, J, Shoam, Z, Rudak, E, Nebel, L, Goldman B and Ben-Rafael, Z (1988). Programmed oocytes retrieval; The concept of programmed cycles. Ann NY Acad Sci. In press

7. Zorn, JR, Boyer, P, and Guichard, A (1987). Programming for IVF-ET and GIFT. Lancet, 1, 385

8. Sheehan, KL, Casper, RF, and Yen, SSC (1982). Induction of luteolysis by luteinizing hormone releasing factor (LRF) agonist: Sensitivity, reproducibility, and reversibility. Fertil Steril, 37, 209

9. Popkin, R, Bramley, TA, Curries, A, Shaw, RW, Baird, DT and Fraser, HM (1983). Specific binding of luteinizing hormone releasing hormone to human luteal tissue. Biohem Biophys Res Commun, 114, 750

5. Cohen, J., Debache, C., Pigeau, F., Mandelbaum, J., Plachot, M. and de Mouzon, J. (1987) ... Results of planned in-vitro fertilization programming through the pre-administration of oestrogen progestogen combined pill. Human Reprod. 2, ...

6. ... Mandelbaum, J., Plachot, M., Junca, A.M., ... [illegible]

7. ... LHRH agonist ... (1988) ... IVF-ET and GIFT ... 3, 203

8. ... Sharma, V., ... (1988) ... Improvement ... of ... luteinizing hormone releasing factor (LHRF) agonist: sensitivity, reproducibility, and ... fertility. Fertil. Steril. ... 201

9. ... Rose, M., ... E., ... and ... (1988) ... of ... ... Human Reprod. ... Contr. 14, 150

18

IMPROVED PREGNANCY RATE IN IVF/ET BY COMBINED LONG-ACTING GnRH ANALOGUE AND GONADOTROPINS

R. RON-EL, E. CASPI, H. NACHUM, A. GOLAN, A. HERMAN, Y. SOFFER and Z. WEINRAUB
Department of Obstetrics and Gynecology, Assaf Harofe Medical Centre, Zerefin Sackler School of Medicine, Tel-Aviv University, Israel

INTRODUCTION

The cancellation rate in In Vitro Fertilization - Embryo Transfer (IVF-Et) programmes of 20-30% [1, 2, 3] has brought us to use a GnRH analogue regimen prior to hMG administration. In order to achieve a satisfactory suppression of the endogenous activity of the hypothalamic-pituitary-ovarian axis, with the convenience of a single injection, we have chosen to use a long acting GnRH analogue preparation. We present here our experience in 143 consecutive treated cycles.

MATERIALS AND METHODS

According to daily hormonal results in 3 menstrual volunteers (D. Ayalon, personal communication) who received D-TRP-6-LH-RH-CR, (Decapeptyl-Microcapsules 3.2mg, Ferring, Kiel, West Germany) and the pharmocokinetics of this preparation (Happ et al, submitted for publication), our treatment protocol was as follows: When no follicles or cysts were ultrasonically demonstrated, a single injection of the above mentioned analogue was administered intramuscularly on the first day of menstruation (day 0). On day 17-18, pituitary suppression was tested by 17ß Estradiol (E_2) Progesterone (P) and LH levels together with ultrasound examination of the ovaries to exclude any remnant cysts. HMG stimulation, initially using 3 ampoules per day, was started when E_2, P and LH levels were lower than 50pg/ml and durations of administration were individually adjusted. HCG (10,000 IU) was administered when serum E_2 was on the rise and the leading follicles reached a diameter of 18mm . An additional 2500 IU of hCG as given every third day during the luteal phase. Oocyte retrieval was generally vaginally guided by ultrasonography. In cases with three or less demonstrated follicles, or both ovaries behind the uterus, laporoscopy was the preferred ovum pick up method.

One hundred and forty three treatment cycles were carried out on 117 patients. The patient selection and clinical

Table 1. Clinical characteristics of the study group.

Cause of Infertility	Total	I° Inf.	II° Inf.
Tubal	43%	36%	64%
Unexplained	43%	74%	26%
Male	8%	-	-
Endometriosis	2%	-	-
Others	4%	-	-

characteristics are shown in Table 1. Of them 43 patients (30%) had at least one previous cancellation because of early luteinization. Their mean age was 31.9± 3.4 years and the duration of infertility was 6.4 ± 4.3 years.

The culture medium used was Earl's B.S.S. (Gibco Cat No.. 041-4015) supplemented with 10% inactivated fetal cord serum. Sperm were prepared by washing and swim-up procedures, and oocyte insemination using 100,000 motile sperms took place 1.7 hours after retrieval. Replacement during the first parts of our programme (prior to freezing) used up to 5 and later up to 4 embryos per transfer. The transfer was performed in the lithotomy position using the Wallace Catheter (No. 18146) in a volume of 30 microliters (90% serum).

RESULTS

The numbers of hMG ampoules used for ovarian hyperstimulation and the distribution of the oocyte retrievals during the week are presented in Table 2. The hormonal profile of the whole study group is shown in Table 3. Of the 143 treated cycles, 4 (2.8%)

Table 2. Ovarian stimulation data.

Parameter	Mean	Range
hMG Ampoules	37.8	11 - 94
hMG Days	11.4	5 - 23
Start of hMG Post Decapeptyl (days)	19.4	16 - 31

Table 3. Hormonal profile on hCG administration day.

Hormone	Mean	SD	Range
2_2	1589	1166	290 - 7180
P	1.1	0.6	0.2 - 3.3
LH	9.1	3.5	2.8 - 26.5

were cancelled because of escaped ovulation. Cyst formation prior to hMG administration occurred in 14 cases (9.8%) and 5 cases (3.5%) were associated with a low response (E_2 on hCG administration day <300pg/ml and/or 2 or less follicles). The mean number of oocytes retrieved, fertilization, cleavage and pregnancy rates are shown in Tables 4 and 5.

Table 4. Outcome of retrieval and fertilization procedures.

Procedure	Outcome
Vaginal Oocyte pickup	105
Laparoscopic Oocyte pickup	34
Cycles with Oocytes	99%
Oocytes per Cycle	7.0
Fertilization Rate	46%
Cleavage Rate	94%
Embryo Transfer Rate	76%

Table 5. End results of procedure.

Procedure	Number (%)
Pregnancy/Cycle	44/143 (31)
Pregnancy/ET	44/105 (42)
Early Abortions	9 (20)
Late Abortions	3 (7)
Multiple Pregnancies	8 (18)
Ovarian Hyperstimulation	12 (8)

In the cyst formation group, when the suppression period was continued and the administration of hMG postponed, the cysts disappeared or became smaller, and the outcome in these cases was within the range of the total study group. In the low response group, on the other hand few oocytes (in one case 5, in 2 cases 2 and in the remaining 2, none) were obtained. Only one pregnancy was achieved in this last group.

The side effects due to the GnRH analogue injection consisted of spotting of uterine blood in 58%, hot flushes in 42%, headache and tiredness in 34%, nausea in 15% of the patients and were limited to the period prior to hMG administration.

DISCUSSION

The use of a GnRH analogue for temporary suppression of the pituitary enables ovarian stimulation without interference from the endogenous pituitary activity. The use of a long acting GnRH preparation (Decapeptyl) gives a continuous and steady state of suppression, with the flexibility to postpone hMG administration individually according to the case. In our study group we delayed hMG administration up to 32 days, still followed by successful conceptual cycles.

The very low cancellation rate (2.8%) due to escaped ovulation is an undoubted merit of the treatment regimen . Our impression is that the relatively high number of oocytes with good morphology achieved (78%) by this combination regimen, probably brings about a syncronised growth of the follicles, and so more embryos are available per cycle treatment. The optimal ranges of the LH and P on the hCG administration day in this series, which are much lower than in the "no conception zone" [4, 5], also add to a better oocyte quality. It is our opinion that the above-mentioned may be the reasons for the relatively better pregnancy rate achieved in this study group compared to previously published studies.

REFERENCES

1. Belaisch-Allart, JC, Frydman, R, Testart, J, Guillet-Rosso, F, Lassale, B, VVolante, M, and Papiernik, F (1984). In vitro fertilization and embryuo transfer program in Clamart, France. J In Vitro Fert Embryo Transfer, 1, 51

2. Van Eum, IFHM, Garcia, JH, Lin, HC, and Rosenwaks, Z (1986). Clinical aspects with regard to the occurence of an endogenous luteinizing hormone surger in gonadotrophin induced normal menstrual cycles. J In Vitro Fert Embryo Transfer, 3, 345-352

3. Trounson, A and Wood, C (1984). In vitro fertilization results 1979-1982 at Monash University, Queen Victoria and Epworth Medical Centres. J In Vitro Fert Embryo Transfer 1, 42

4. Howles, Cm, MacNamee, MC, and Walters, DE (1987). Tonic levels of luteinizing hormone and the outcome of IVF. Human Reproduction, Abstracts from the 3rd meeting of the European Society of Human Reproduction and Embryology, p. 19, June 28-July 1, Cambridge

5. Yovich, JL, McColm, SC, Yovich, JM, and Matson, PL (1985). Early luteal serum progesterone concentrations are higher in pregnancy cycles. Fertil Steril, 44, 184

INDEX